Robert Priest is Professor of Psychiatry at the University of London, and Honorary Consultant at St Mary's Hospital in London.

During more than thirty-five years of specialized research and patient care, he has won, among many other international distinctions, the A. E. Bennett Award from the United States Society for Biological Psychiatry, and the Gutheil Von Domarus Award from the Association for the Advancement of Psychotherapy and American Journal of Psychotherapy, New York.

He has been President of the Society for Psychosomatic Research, and a Member of the Council of the British Association for Psychopharmacology. He was Vice-President of the International College of Psychosomatic Medicine, Registrar of the Royal College of Psychiatrists, and Chairman of the Mental Health Group in the British Medical Association. He was recently Senator and Chairman of the Board of Studies in Medicine at the University of London.

Professor Priest is a member of the editorial boards of a number of specialist journals and is author of over 200 scientific articles. He is well known around the world and has lectured widely in North and South America, Australia, Europe, the Middle East and Asia.

Professor Priest is married with two sons and, in what little spare time is left to him, keeps active with squash, tennis, jogging and swimming.

D0488934

ANXIETY AND DEPRESSION

A practical guide to recovery

Robert Priest

MD, FRCP (Edinburgh), FRCPsych

VERMILION
LONDON

First published by Martin Dunitz Limited in 1983

5 7 9 10 8 6 4

Copyright © Robert G. Priest 1983

Robert G. Priest has asserted his moral right to be identified as the author of this work in accordance with the Copyright, Design and Patents Act 1988.

All rights reserved. No part of this publication may be reproduced, stored in a retrieval system, or transmitted in any form or by any means, electronic, mechanical, photocopying, recording or otherwise, without the prior permission of the copyright owner.

This edition published in the United Kingdom in 1996 by Vermillion an imprint of Ebury Press

Random House UK Ltd
Random House
20 Vauxhall Bridge Road
London SW1V 2SA

Random House Australia (Pty) Ltd
20 Alfred Street, Milsons Point, Sydney,
New South Wales 2061, Australia

Random House New Zealand Limited
18 Poland Road, Glenfield,
Auckland 10, New Zealand

Random House, South Africa (Pty) Limited
PO Box 337, Bergvlei, South Africa

The Random House Group Limited Reg. No. 954009

www.randomhouse.co.uk

A CIP catalogue record for this book is available from the British Library.

ISBN 0 09 181266 6

Typeset in Times Roman by Deltatype Ltd, Ellesmere Port, Cheshire
Printed and bound in Great Britain by Mackays of Chatham, plc.

Papers used by Vermilion are natural, recyclable products made from wood grown in sustainable forests.

To David, Carol, Christopher and Melanie

CONTENTS

ACKNOWLEDGMENTS

I am very indebted to Douglas for his practical assistance in the preparation of this book. I am deeply grateful to Marilyn for her sympathetic encouragement and understanding counselling, and to Ursula for her perceptive suggestions and expert help.

The case histories in the book are based on clinical experience but neither they nor the names relate to any particular individual.

Robert Priest, London 1983

We are grateful to Jane Madders who advised on the massage and relaxation techniques.

The diagrams on pages 6, 17, 83 and 108 were drawn by Cathy Clench. The diagrams on pages 6 and 17 are derived from information published by G. A. Foulds and K. Hope. The diagram on page 108 is derived from information published by Stewart Agras, MD, David Sylvester, PhD, and Donald Oliveau, MD, in *Comprehensive Psychiatry*, Vol 10 No 2 (March), 1969. All other illustrations by Peter Cox.

Finally, thanks are due to Jennifer Eaton, BSc, MSc, MPS, for information on international drug-name equivalents.

INTRODUCTION

Anxiety and depression are normal parts of our lives. Few of us have not felt anxious or depressed at some time, and the causes are often obvious. We all have disappointments and losses to face; we all have fears and uncertainties. I shall explain how major changes in our lives – like becoming a parent or retiring – can cause unpleasant feelings of all kinds.

However, anxiety and depression can be serious – even life-threatening – problems, and it is only in recent years that doctors have focused their attention on them as illnesses which can be treated. It is now thought that millions of people all over the world suffer from anxiety and depression to such an extent that it makes leading a normal life difficult. Estimates vary, but it seems likely that at least 10 per cent of the populations of developed Western countries suffer from them seriously enough to need help – and some experts have put the figure as high as 30 per cent. That means at least 20 million people in the United States alone.

Unfortunately many people still think that anxiety and depression are not real illnesses. If you are feeling anxious or depressed, you might have found other people to be unsympathetic or even hostile. You will know, however, that being told to 'snap out of it' does no good whatsoever. You need to know what is happening to you; and you may need help.

It is also difficult for many people to admit openly that they are suffering from an emotional problem like this. As you will see, anxiety or depression – and the unpleasant emotional and physical symptoms they cause – can be very mystifying. You may begin to worry that you are going mad, especially if those around you seem to misunderstand your feelings.

It was encountering precisely these problems as a family doctor – the uncertainties and the mysterious nature of anxiety and depression – that originally fired my interest in this field and led me to specialize in psychiatry in the early 1960s. Today, as well as carrying out research into the causes and treatments of emotional problems, I see a large number of patients each year, of whom around 80 per cent suffer from anxiety or depression. I hope this book will communicate some of the insight I have gained into these conditions over the last thirty years, and help to clear up the mystery that continues to surround them.

I believe that many anxious men and women do not need to suffer so much. They are not insane, and they can be helped. Your burden can be lifted and shared, and your distress relieved. In the vast majority of cases, people with even quite severe anxiety or depression can be helped to live normal lives again. This book is also aimed at people who are trying to help a loved one, a relative or friend overcome anxiety or depression. If you are in this position, you may find that learning in the book about the way doctors, psychiatrists, therapists and other specialists treat their anxious and depressed patients will provide you with ideas and guidelines on how you yourself can help. I have also included sections that give practical advice specially for the sufferer's family and friends. I hope that more and more people will come to recognize these problems for what they are – and that as a result, more sufferers will gain the support or treatment they need. It is sad that very often people with anxiety or depression may not get any real assistance until they have suffered for far too long.

In the course of this book, I shall explain what anxiety and depression are, what causes them and how they affect you. I shall be offering advice on how you can help yourself to overcome them, and also when it is time to seek professional help. I will describe what it is like to feel so upset that you are unable to cope with your day-to-day life. You will find out how you can be treated when you have reached this stage – and what sort of treatment is best for your particular problem.

Before we go any further, it is important for you to remember one thing. Even if you feel so tense or downhearted that everything seems hopeless, do not despair. Almost always, things get better in time. I hope that this book will help you (or your loved one) towards a speedy and lasting recovery.

1
WHAT IS ANXIETY?

Anxiety or 'feeling anxious' is something we all talk about from time to time. As with most words we use to describe our feelings and emotions, anxiety can refer to many different things in many different circumstances. Before we can look at how to cope with anxiety, we need to find out what the things we experience have in common. This will also help us to understand how anxiety is linked to depression, the subject of my next chapter.

The first two things to understand are that anxiety can cover a broad range of experiences, and that it can be completely normal even when it is extreme. For example, you might feel mildly anxious about starting a new job; and you will certainly feel very anxious indeed if someone you love has been involved in an accident and is critically ill.

There we have two examples of anxiety, one mild and one severe. But no one would think they were extreme or out of proportion in the circumstances. It might be distressing for your friends to see you so worried in the second example, and even puzzling for your more confident friends to see you worried about a new job – something they would take in their stride. But your reactions in both situations would be normal.

What do these two examples have in common? They both involve feelings about something which you think might be going to happen. Before you arrive at your new job you might worry about whether you are going to enjoy it or get on with your colleagues. You will not know until you actually start the job. In the example of being worried about someone who is critically ill, you will probably be afraid that they might die or be severely handicapped.

One of the best definitions of anxiety I have heard is that it is 'fear spread out thin'. Anxiety is the feeling you have when you think that something unpleasant is going to happen in the future. You might use other words and phrases to describe it, saying that you are feeling 'apprehensive', 'uncertain', 'nervous', 'wound up', 'on edge' or that you are 'dreading the worst'.

THE STRESSES AND UNCERTAINTIES OF LIFE

A certain amount of anxiety is the price we pay for living a normal life. Life is full of stresses and uncertainties: cars that will not start, bills which have to be paid, illnesses of all kinds, from mild colds to life-threatening conditions. We all have problems to face occasionally, and being human means that we can see problems coming, sometimes a long time before they arrive.

Common sources of anxiety

- Relationships
- Health
- Your children
- Pregnancy
- Growing old

- Your job
- Promotion
- Financial difficulties
- Legal problems
- Exams

- Domestic upheaval

It might be easier if we think of anxiety as a response to a threat, real or imagined. It can be a physical threat which causes anxiety; a child who thinks he might be bullied at school is likely to feel apprehensive at the prospect. Or the threat might be more abstract. The same child might feel very anxious about an examination if he knows his parents are very keen for him to do well at school. He fears their disapproval if he fails.

In this sense of responding to a threat, anxiety can sometimes be an advantage. That child's anxiety might make him take action to stop the bullying by telling his parents, for example. The unpleasantness of the feeling makes him want it to be taken away. His anxiety about the examination might make him more attentive in class, too, so that he strives for the best possible performance in the test itself.

Quite often your anxiety may spur you on to make decisions, take steps, engage in practical activities to find solutions. A threat is posed, your attention is concentrated, and you meet it. But difficulties can arise when either you cannot find a solution or your anxiety is out of proportion to the circumstances. But before we look at these, it will be helpful if you can recognize the ways in which your body reacts to anxiety.

HOW YOUR BODY MAY REACT TO ANXIETY

So far I have been talking about what goes on in your mind when you feel anxious. Most feelings have their physical side too, and anxiety is no exception.

1. **Palpitations** When you are under stress you might feel your heart racing and pounding.

2. **Shaking** You may find that you are shaking or trembling, especially if you have had a shock or are upset. Either your hands shake when you try to do something, or your knees wobble. You might have butterflies in the stomach or shake all over. These are all signs of fear.

3. **Tension** One of the best known signs of anxiety is tension. You might feel that the muscles of the back of your neck are very tight and tense, and this produces pain. Tension in the muscles of the scalp is one of the causes of headaches which accompany worry. You might also feel that the tension is not in a specific place, but is just a vague feeling, a sense that you are strung up and cannot relax.

4. **Insomnia** Often sleep is affected. You may have difficulty getting to sleep, and even when you finally drop off, you might be restless and wake up several times during the night. Your dreams might be vivid and turn into nightmares, and you will probably wake up in the morning feeling tired and unrefreshed.

5. **Perspiration** Some people find that anxiety makes them sweat excessively, even on cool days.

6. **Other physical signs** of anxiety and tension can be nausea, numbness, tingling in the hands and feet and a desire to urinate more often than usual.

All these physical signs of anxiety are related to the so-called 'fight or

Symptoms of anxiety

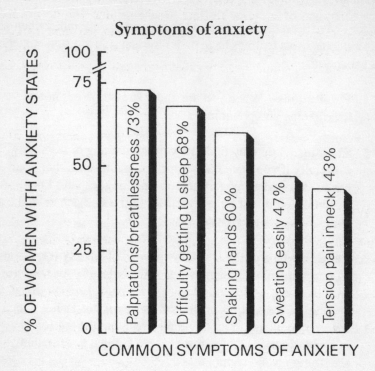

Based on a survey of women suffering from anxiety, this shows how commonly the different physical symptoms are experienced.

flight' instinct we have inherited from our prehistoric ancestors. The sort of threats they faced in their daily lives were most probably physical – being attacked by other people or wild animals, for example.

Their bodies reacted to threat by preparing themselves for action, either fighting or running away. The heart beats faster to provide more blood for using the muscles, and sweating helps to cool the skin during vigorous movement and exercise. The muscles are tensed and prepared to respond, and if they are held in this state for too long they will begin to ache.

This was the way our ancestors prepared themselves to deal with physical threats. Our bodies' responses to danger are no different now, although, as we have seen, the sorts of threats and problems we have to face today are often quite abstract. Realizing that you do not have enough money to pay several large bills is not the same as being frightened by a dangerous animal. But it still poses a danger, and your body reacts in a similar way, to protect yourself or your loved ones.

WHEN ANXIETY GETS OUT OF PROPORTION

So anxiety has two parts which go together, an emotional and a physical reaction. Being anxious about something might become a problem when you find that it is out of proportion – when you find you are feeling much more anxious than you would expect someone to be in your circumstances.

This is easier to grasp if we look at one particular example. Students often feel anxious before exams, and this is quite understandable. This anxiety helps to sharpen the mind and focus it on the task in hand, that is, getting through the exam. We might say that a student had a problem if he found himself paralysed with anxiety months ahead. He himself might become very worried if he was not sleeping well and had some of the other physical symptoms we have described. In this case he will probably need some assistance to overcome the anxiety, because it is no longer a help in sharpening his response, but a hindrance. The anxiety will get in the way and make life more difficult.

The same is true of any anxiety. If you are anxious about something which you cannot resolve, and which continues to hang over you, then you will feel all the more tense until the tension itself becomes a problem. This could be the beginning of a vicious circle, with anxiety making more difficulties, which then cause further anxiety, and so on. We will be looking at ways you can break out of this circle of anxiety in Chapter 3.

Severe anxiety

In these terms, anxiety is something we can all understand. But anxiety can be particularly disturbing when you experience it for no obvious reason. Most of us are anxious about certain things, like taking exams, starting new jobs, our health, money, relationships with those near to us. But as we handle difficult situations we gain experience, and each success – however minor – leads to a growth in our confidence. Success breeds success, and we find that we become less anxious about new challenges. Some people seem to be prone to anxiety as a way of life, even if they obviously cope with problems successfully. Basically, they lack self-confidence, and there can be many causes of this. One could be that they were brought up to believe they were less capable than they really are, so each challenge brings back memories of parents being negative about their potential success. It is also true that some people only succeed by becoming extremely anxious about their careers, especially where they are faced with tough competition. If you are like this, then it might be quite easy to see where the anxiety is coming from.

If you lack self-confidence, as in the first example, it might be that you just need a little more time than others to gain the confidence to handle life, but that will come in the end. If professional pressure makes you continually anxious, as in the second example, you might thrive on 'brinkmanship', but if you do not, the answer may be simple – changing to a less demanding career, perhaps.

Many people can suffer from seemingly inexplicable attacks of anxiety from time to time without any obvious threat in their lives. The attacks can be terrifying, especially as there appears to be no cause for them. These people may have much higher levels of anxiety than 'normal' between attacks, too. In this case doctors would probably say they were suffering from an anxiety state. A general feeling of anxiety – with physical symptoms and no obvious cause – which never seems to go away is called 'free-floating' anxiety.

Someone who feels continually anxious will begin to suffer emotionally and physically, whether or not there is an obvious cause. We have seen what the physical symptoms of anxiety are; if these are experienced over a long period, they can affect your health, your mental state and your family, friends and colleagues.

As we shall see, if people who suffer in this way are not helped, they can slip into depression – and even have physical illnesses. Heart disease is a case in point. It has been shown that although other factors – such as diet and lack of exercise – can play a large part in heart and circulation problems, stress and anxiety are major causes of them.

If your heart beats at an abnormally high rate for years because of your anxiety, and your blood pressure is high and the blood vessels therefore narrowed, then you are at a much higher risk of having a heart attack or stroke. Other disorders like stomach ulcers have also been linked with stress, and there has been much comment by doctors about the link between our stress- (and anxiety-) ridden society and the rise in the number of people suffering from these disorders.

These are serious results of long-term stress and anxiety, and show the importance of doing something about them before the situation becomes this bad.

PHOBIAS

Phobias are also related to stress and anxiety. They differ in two ways from the anxiety we have been discussing so far. First, rather than being vague fears of future events, they are fears of specific objects or situations. And second, they are not 'spread out thin', but excessive, out of proportion to their circumstances, and can totally disrupt your normal way of life.

Many people are frightened of snakes, but if you became so terrified of them that you refused to walk along streets even in areas or countries where there are no harmful species, then you would have a phobia. That is, your life would be made difficult by your fear.

Often a phobia disguises other underlying problems and is just the tip of the iceberg. It is also true that a seemingly inexplicable anxiety can be caused by a phobia. For example, if a woman begins to suffer from the physical signs of anxiety every time she goes shopping, she may be mystified. But it could be that she has developed one of the commonest forms of phobia to affect women, agoraphobia – often thought to be a fear of open spaces. In fact it is not as simple as that. Many housewives with agoraphobia feel panicky at the thought of having to go to the local supermarket to do their shopping. The word 'agoraphobia' means literally 'fear of the market place'.

I shall be looking at phobias in detail in Chapter 9. Suffice it to say here that it is thought they are often the result of one extreme anxiety-provoking situation in early life that leaves an 'emotional scar'. If you have an excessive fear of snakes, it might be that as a child you saw or were even bitten by one in terrifying circumstances. The anxiety you felt then remains with you, perhaps becoming worse at times of stress or if you come into contact with snakes again.

PHYSICAL CAUSES OF ANXIETY

One other important point to make is that anxiety can sometimes be caused by an illness. An overactive thyroid gland, for example, will produce the symptoms of anxiety – and if you have the physical symptoms, you may feel anxious, even when there is no apparent cause.

Some other physical illnesses can also lead to the physical symptoms of anxiety, so it is vital to make sure that there is nothing bodily wrong with you. We will look at the tests your doctor can perform to rule out physical illness as a cause of anxiety in Chapter 4. Giving up cigarettes, alcohol, or even certain types of sleeping pill can cause anxiety if you have been taking them for an extended period and have become dependent on them. Again, if the problem is severe, you may need help from your doctor.

HOW COMMON IS ANXIETY?

It is difficult to say exactly how many people suffer from anxiety. First, because a certain amount of anxiety is normal in everyone's life; and second, because it only becomes a problem that might be taken to a doctor or specialist when it begins to affect someone's ability to lead a 'normal' life, and there must be a vast number of people who would benefit from treatment but who continue to struggle on without seeking help.

Nonetheless, we do know that anxiety is very common. It seems to be slightly more common in women than men (around twice as many women than men actually seek help for anxiety). In one survey I conducted in Britain, I found that of all the people going to their family doctors with emotional problems, more than half were suffering from anxiety. And of all the patients I see, over 70 per cent report anxiety as one of their symptoms. Remember too that it can happen to anyone at any time in life.

I shall examine ways in which you can cope with anxiety in Chapter 3, and how people with severe anxiety can be helped, in later chapters. First, though, let's see what happens when that dreaded future event arrives and depression sets in.

2
WHAT IS
DEPRESSION?

Depression is similar to anxiety in many ways, and the two are linked. Depression is an emotion with a strong physical side. It can often come after a period of anxiety, be caused by anxiety or go hand in hand with it. In fact, around 80 per cent of sufferers from either anxiety or depression are affected by both together.

Where it differs from anxiety is that it is generally caused by something that has already happened. In our example of feeling nervous before starting a new job, if you found you hated it once you had started, then it would be quite normal to feel depressed. It would be a bitter blow, especially if you had hoped for great things from that particular job. And if you explained the position to your family and friends, they would understand – your depression would be normal in the circumstances. You get the feeling of depression when something bad has definitely happened to you (or you know for certain that it's going to) – and that is the simplest definition of depression there is.

Of course, in our example of a loved one who is critically ill, depression could play a part too. If it was a long illness, the weight of anxiety might make you feel very low. If your loved one died, then depression would again be normal; indeed, those around you would be surprised if you did not show any of the 'appropriate' emotions. In those circumstances we have a very familiar word for this situation and its feelings – grief. I shall be taking a closer look at bereavement in Chapter 3.

In these senses, depression is an everyday experience. We are all depressed from time to time, and we have many ways of describing the feeling. You can be 'fed up', 'down in the dumps', 'blue', 'unhappy', 'sad', 'down-hearted' or 'low'. Depression can last for a few minutes or a few days or longer, and is often the result of some kind of loss: loss of a relative, of a relationship, of your good health, of money, status, freedom, and many other important things besides. You can also sometimes become depressed about something which has not happened yet: when you know something unpleasant is inevitable, like losing your job or a loved one.

STRESS AND DEPRESSION

Another similarity between anxiety and depression is that they are both in some ways essential parts of being human. Life is full of stresses, and that means that it can also be full of disappointments and unresolved problems.

We all have a store of things in our pasts which we sometimes feel unhappy about. For some people these things are minor: being jilted, or making a mistake at work. For others they might be more major: a terrible disappointment, losing a spouse at a crucial stage, failure of a business, and so on.

Common sources of depression

- Unhappy relationships
- Parenthood
- Divorce/separation
- Children leaving home
- Financial difficulties

- Redundancy
- Retirement
- Old age
- Illness
- Bereavement

- Failure at work

Most of us overcome our feelings of depression and manage to recover our emotional equilibrium. As with anxiety, sometimes a period of depression can be productive; it can make us think about past failures or disappointments and consider how we might take steps to avoid similar disappointments in future.

Grief itself can be seen as a protective reaction too, just like certain types of anxiety. It is a way of retreating from the world at a time when the mind needs to cope with a massive and upsetting change. If anxiety focuses the mind and body on a coming threat, then depression focuses the mind and body inwards, on recovery, on a general thinking out and adaptation to a change in circumstances brought about by a major event.

WHEN DEPRESSION GETS OUT OF PROPORTION

Depression, like anxiety, becomes a problem when it gets out of proportion. We understand that someone might feel a little depressed after a minor disappointment, but we would begin to feel it was not normal if the depression after a trivial event was either very severe or went on for too long.

The same is true of more serious depressions. If someone becomes completely broken up by grief after a loved one's death, that falls within the range of what we would consider 'normal'. But if that depression is still incapacitating months or even years later, then we might feel that it had got out of hand and that some sort of help was needed.

In the end, deciding when a depression – whether it is ours or somebody else's – is abnormal is a very difficult decision in many cases. As with anxiety, the best guideline is that when depression begins to take over your life and affect everything adversely, then you may well need help. But before we look at severe, disabling depression, we need to find out how to recognize the symptoms.

THE PSYCHOLOGICAL SYMPTOMS

It is important to remember that you might not experience all the following symptoms together. You might feel more sad than anything else, or it might be a loss of energy which distresses you most. But the majority of people who are badly depressed will experience most of these symptoms during their depression, some more strongly than others.

It is also true that some people have very few symptoms of depression at all and yet are still feeling very low, while others may feel them and not be suffering from a serious depression at all. With this in mind, it is wise to remember the following rule of thumb. If you are experiencing three or more of these symptoms – particularly the sadness and the morbid thoughts – then you may well need help.

1. **Sadness** The commonest, and most obvious, symptom of depression is sadness. This melancholy is likely to be persistent, and it might be accompanied by a tendency to cry more often

than usual, even at the slightest upset – or without any upset at all.

2. **Loss of interest**   When you are depressed you will probably lose interest in most things, even your favourite pastimes. You will not wish to read the paper, or watch television, you cease to care about your hobbies, or your job.

3. **Loss of energy**   Along with this loss of interest will go a loss of energy. Everything seems to be a great effort and too much trouble, even minor things, like taking care of your personal appearance and hygiene.

4. **Loss of concentration**   Concentration becomes difficult, and you might find yourself reading the same line in a book over and over again without remembering it. You may also tend to forget things and become absent-minded.

5. **Morbid thoughts**   Depression turns your mind to depressing things, and you might find yourself thinking for no reason that you have a serious illness like cancer. You might begin to worry about every little thing and become very pessimistic.

6. **Guilt**   Another typical symptom is guilt. Depressed people sometimes have an overwhelming belief that they are guilty of terrible crimes, even if the so-called crimes seem very minor to other people.

7. **Unworthiness**   Allied to the feelings of guilt are feelings of unworthiness. You might feel that you are unworthy of any help or sympathy in your predicament, and many depressed people tend to lose their self-respect.

THE PHYSICAL SYMPTOMS

Again, as with the psychological symptoms of depression, you may not experience all the following symptoms together, and some may be more serious than others. Sleep disturbances and constipation, for example, may give you more distress than any of the others.

Follow the same rule of thumb: if three or more of these symptoms are affecting you, it might be time to ask yourself if you are depressed and if you need a change in life-style or some help.

1. **Loss of appetite** People often go off their food when they are feeling depressed, and this might lead to a large loss in weight in someone who is severely depressed. Some people, though, overeat instead.

2. **Sleep disturbances** As with people suffering from anxiety, depression might make it difficult for you to get off to sleep in the first place. Afterwards your sleep might be broken by wakeful, restless spells. Severely depressed people are particularly prone to early morning waking. You might wake up very early and not be able to get back to sleep. And you may well find that this is the time of day when your spirits are at their lowest ebb.

3. **Slowing down** This is part of the loss of energy we have already talked about. Actions like walking and talking feel slow and difficult, and often somebody watching a depressed person can see that they actually are slowed up.

4. **Constipation** The slowing down may even affect parts of your body which are not under the conscious control of the mind, like the intestine. Depressed people can become so constipated that they begin to think they must have a more serious bowel condition.

5. **Loss of sex drive** Both men and women can go off sex while they are depressed, and this in itself can increase their feelings of depression and inadequacy.

6. **Other symptoms** Headaches, backaches and pains in the face and neck are also quite common in depression. People who are suffering from a mixture of anxiety and depression may have some or all of the symptoms we looked at in Chapter 1, as well.

TWO TYPES OF DEPRESSION

These symptoms are easily explained when you have suffered a disappointment. If we take loss of interest and loss of energy, for example, there is a very simple way of explaining them. We all have more enthusiasm and energy for jobs we want to do. When you are going up a flight of stairs, you will probably find it easier to go up if you are expecting to enjoy what is at the top. You may even run up two at a time!

If you are not looking forward to what is at the top, it will be much more exhausting to go up these same stairs. You might drag yourself up, one stair at a time. Your legs will ache, and it will all seem to be a great effort. You generally have more energy for those activities which you are interested in, so it makes sense that when you lose your interest in something you lose the energy to do it.

In depression, the explanation is not always so obvious. These symptoms are understandable when you know what is causing your feelings of depression. They are much more mystifying – and probably more worrying – if there appears to be no cause. Depressions like this, which seem to come from 'within', are called endogenous (meaning literally 'created within'). Depressions which have an obvious cause are called reactive.

We shall see in Chapter 3 that the cause of your depression – like the cause of your anxiety – has an important part to play in how you cope with it and eventually overcome it. We will also see in Chapter 7 that specialist help might be needed if your depression is related to deeper problems in your feelings and approach to life.

SEVERE DEPRESSION

Depression can become severe, whether it is reactive or endogenous – in other words, whether there is an obvious external cause or not. The symptoms we have already looked at become worse or grow in number, and if you are very depressed, you might begin to feel that there is no way out. That feeling in itself is likely to lead to even more depression, and as with anxiety, the more hopeless you feel, the worse you can get, and so on, in a downward vicious circle. People who reach this stage are said by doctors to be suffering from a depressive illness.

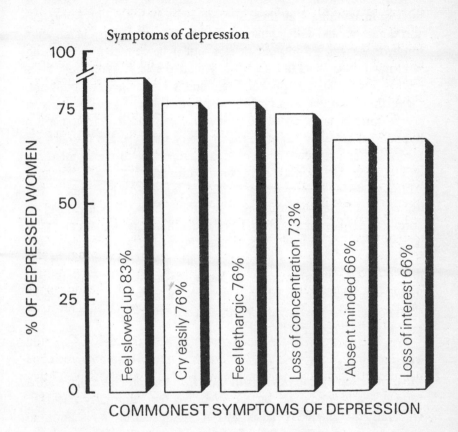

Symptoms of depression

% OF DEPRESSED WOMEN

100
75
50
25
0

Feel slowed up 83%
Cry easily 76%
Feel lethargic 76%
Loss of concentration 73%
Absent minded 66%
Loss of interest 66%

COMMONEST SYMPTOMS OF DEPRESSION

Based on a survey of women suffering from depression, this shows how commonly some of the different symptoms are experienced.

It is very difficult to break this vicious circle on your own. If you are left to yourself when you are feeling severely depressed, you might tend to think of unpleasant things, feel pessimistic about everything and generally make yourself feel worse. In the early stages of a depression, you might seek out your friends for help and sympathy. But if there is no obvious reason for your feelings, they might not prove to be very sympathetic; and if your depression deepens, whether there is any cause or not, you might begin to avoid people and sink into isolation – which will not do you any good at all.

Absent-mindedness, loss of concentration and energy, a lack of interest in anything – all these symptoms make it difficult for you to sort things out and help yourself to feel better. Your physical ailments might make you go to your doctor, but if he cannot find anything wrong with you – and fails to detect your depression – you might only begin to feel like a hypochondriac, and your feelings of guilt and unworthiness might seemingly be confirmed. Feeling guilty that you are making a nuisance of yourself, and convinced that you are a hypochondriac, you might begin to worry that you are losing your sanity. After all, what else could be happening to cause all these strange thoughts, morbid feelings and sadness?

The problem is that when a severe depression like this is left untreated, the person suffering from it can finally reach a level of complete despair. In this state, he or she will not be able to cope with life, and career, relationships and health may all begin to break down. Escape may come in the form of alcoholism or some other form of drug abuse. But the ultimate resort for those who feel life is completely unbearable is suicide, and this is a real risk for the severely depressed. I shall be showing how severe depression is treated – and suicide can be avoided – in Chapter 10.

Manic-depressive illness

Most of us have minor swings in mood, so that on one day we are a little down-hearted, and on the next we feel unusually cheerful. Generally this change is caused by our circumstances and is a normal variation in the way we feel. This should not be confused with the extremes of mood experienced by someone who is manic depressive.

Although the term 'manic depressive' is widely known, it is a rare state, affecting only a small percentage of those who suffer from depression.

The manic depressive's life fluctuates between periods of deep depression and euphoric elation that are unrelated to external events. During the manic phase the sufferer becomes wildly excited, cheerful, talkative and restless, often dreaming up extravagant plans, for which he has totally inadequate financial resources.

These violent mood swings are impossible for close friends and family to miss, and it is vital to be aware that a manic-depressive illness is a serious disorder that needs urgent medical attention. It is more complicated and traumatic than straightforward anxiety or depression and really lies outside the scope of this book.

PHYSICAL CAUSES OF DEPRESSION

As with anxiety, it is important to remember that some people's depression has a purely physical cause.

1. **Illness** Just as an overactive thyroid gland can cause anxiety, depression can be caused by a malfunction in other important glands, including the adrenal glands. Depression can also follow certain illnesses like glandular fever – a virus infection which can sometimes leave you feeling low for months afterwards. A bout of flu can do the same. In Chapter 4 we shall see how your doctor will try to find out if there is a physical cause for your depression.

2. **Women's problems** Certain physical aspects of every woman's life can lead to both anxiety and depression. Many women suffer from premenstrual tension (PMT), which can include symptoms of both anxiety and depression. Childbirth too is often followed by mild or serious feelings of being low – something better known as postnatal or postpartum depression. We shall be looking at these problems – and others relating to women – in Chapter 8.

3. **Drugs** Some drugs can make you feel depressed, esecially those used for reducing high blood pressure. If you are taking any course of drugs over a period of time, it is worth asking your doctor about any possible side-effects.

HOW COMMON IS DEPRESSION?

As with anxiety, it is difficult to know exactly how many people suffer from depression. Many people are depressed for short periods or longer ones and get over it. Many people's depression is quite normal in their circumstances, and they eventually get over it, too.

We do know, however, that just like anxiety, depression which is bad enough to make people seek help is very common indeed. It can happen to anyone at any age, but it seems that depression is more likely to occur around crucial times of life such as during puberty – the transition from childhood to adulthood – the early years of being a parent, the menopause, and retirement. These events are laden with stress, and where there is stress there is also likely to be anxiety, and its partner, depression. I shall be dealing with some of these areas in detail in later chapters.

In the survey I conducted of people going to their family doctors because of emotional problems, I found that around 80 per cent were likely to be suffering from depression (many of these of course were experiencing both anxiety and depression). Again, as with anxiety, remember that there are many who would benefit from help. No one has to – or should – suffer severe depression in silence.

3
SELF-HELP WAYS OF OVERCOMING ANXIETY AND DEPRESSION

COPING WITH THE PROBLEMS OF EVERYDAY LIFE

Now that we understand a little more about anxiety and depression, one thing is obvious above all. Life itself is the ultimate cause of emotional problems like these; being alive, having relationships, having to work and strive, bring up children, grow old, retire and to contemplate death, all these things can provoke anxiety and depression. And some of you might be forgiven for thinking that there is little you can do about it; anxiety and depression must seem inevitable.

In a sense this is perfectly true. Anxiety and depression can be normal parts of everybody's life. All the same, they are unpleasant feelings, even when they are minor and short-lived, and everyone would like to avoid them as much as they can and minimize their effects when they occur. We have also seen that when anxiety and depression are not controlled they can set up a vicious circle and then become unnecessarily severe. This is certainly something that can and should be avoided. So in this chapter we are going to look at some positive, practical steps you can take when you are feeling anxious or depressed.

Positive action

Common sense is based on the combined experience of generations of human beings who have lived through many of the difficulties you might be facing now. People have suffered from anxiety and depression since ancient times, and, as you would expect, there are many common-sense approaches to dealing with them. There is also an instinctive side to your responses to them which is worth looking at.

We have already seen how anxiety is a response to a threat, real or imagined. Anxiety itself is part of its own solution; if the anxiety galvanizes you into action, you might overcome the root cause or avoid it. Let's imagine that you are worried about money. You are so worried that you cannot get to sleep at night, your head aches and your heart beats like a drum when you get a letter from your bank. If all this focuses your attention on the crisis, it might help you to start sorting things out. You might see where you can make economies, or how you can earn more money. By doing these things you overcome the threat and relieve your anxiety.

Admittedly life is not always quite so simple. You might not be able to save any money, and if you have just lost your job then things could be very difficult indeed. The thing to remember is that for many people there are solutions, even temporary or unwelcome ones, and that anxiety in particular is a signal that you need to start thinking about your way of life to see if there is something wrong.

Remember too that anxiety and depression might make the right action difficult to take. People who find themselves burdened with money problems sometimes opt for the 'flight' part of the 'fight or flight' instinct and run away from their troubles either metaphorically or literally. This is not usually a real solution; but very often it is difficult to see exactly what the right solution is. It can be very hard to stand back from your life and try to work out objectively what you need to do to sort yourself out – but it is possible.

Taking a vacation Positive action is often a great help in dealing with the causes of anxiety, but sometimes it is more difficult to overcome depression in this way. After all, the cause of your depression is likely to be in the past, so there may not be much you can do about it. One common-sense solution, however, is to take a break.

This can be as short as an evening out or as long as a full vacation: either will do if it takes your mind off what's troubling you and gives you a lift. This sort of self-help can be very successful, especially with mild cases of depression. A break will help to improve your general well-being, and to relax and get over your depression.

Of course it might not be any help at all. If you find yourself sitting on a beach watching everyone else enjoy themselves, unable to join in or relax, then it might make you feel worse. Even if this happens, a vacation might still have its advantages. You might get over the feeling in a couple of days, and if you do not, then it is an important sign that you do need some extra help.

Family and friends Common sense also says that the support of friends and family is an important part of overcoming anxiety and depression in their early stages. Take our previous example of finding out that you hate a new job. Talking it over with your partner or a close friend might help you to see things in perspective. Do you have to stay in the job? Is there something you can do to make it better, like seeing your boss and talking it over? Is there a way of working out the problem which will mean you can stay there?

A friendly, sympathetic ear is a valuable thing to have around. If you are anxious and depressed, opening up about your feelings to somebody else might just clarify them for you, and allow you to see what you need to do.

You might not feel like seeing anyone at all when you're depressed, but it is important to make an effort not to cut yourself off from other people. Just a short chat may be all that's needed to put a rosier hue on life. Low spirits, of course, won't be lifted by those who are unsympathetic and critical, so try to avoid these types of acquaintances if you can.

How to help someone who is anxious or depressed

Few of us are so self-sufficient that we can do everything alone. It is important to realize, therefore, that when someone you know is depressed or anxious they might need help.

How you recognize that they need help – and how you give it – might well be difficult enough. As we have seen, people with anxiety and depression often think that something other than an emotional problem is wrong with them. They might concentrate on their physical ailments or their insomnia, for example, and refuse to talk over their underlying problems. But it you are close enough to someone to know something is wrong, it is time to offer your services as a sympathetic listener. It's important to remember that the person who is suffering might find it difficult to accept your sympathy, understanding, reassurance and advice at first. You should carry on though as you will probably be able to help in the end.

Helping people through grief is a good example of how to go about this. There is nothing you can do to bring somebody back to life, and ignoring the subject is not going to be much help either. If someone you know is depressed after the death of a loved one, they may not want to talk about it at first, but come round to feeling they want to bare their souls later. If you have said that when they want to talk you are ready to listen, you will be doing the best thing possible. The talking itself is their best therapy; it will help them to work through their feelings, get them out in the open, and find a way of getting used to life in a changed form.

One thing which will definitely not help is telling someone to 'snap out of it' or 'pull yourself together'. That is exactly what someone who is tense or feeling low cannot do – it is part of their problem. If they could, they would! One example of how this sort of approach can be counterproductive comes from my own experience.

Mary, a patient of mine, was a forty-three-year-old housewife who totally neglected her housework and allowed her home to become dirty and messy. Her husband realized something was seriously wrong when he found a lot of dirty clothes stuffed under the mattress. He thought his wife was lazy. Being depressed, she felt she was unworthy, and agreed with him. But no amount of telling her not to be lazy was going to help; her problem was more deep-rooted, and turned out in the end to have had a lot to do with her husband's unsympathetic attitude towards her.

Relationships

It is clear from Mary's story that relationships often play a part in anxiety and depression. In fact, one classic definition of the two problems is that anxiety is what happens to you when you think you might lose your lover, depression is what happens after he or she leaves you!

Most people are surrounded by people – lovers, friends, family – and everybody has relationships with those around them. People often play the most important part in our lives and they have the greatest power to give pleasure or inflict suffering on us. The more important someone is to you, then the more able that person is to make you feel anxious or depressed.

Relationships are a fact of life; it would not be wise to avoid them just to prevent the pain they might cause, so the only way to minimize anxiety and depression in your relationships is to look at your attitudes to them. There is a lot to be said for being as open and as honest as you can in your relationships. Not saying what you feel can cause resentments; brooding on past slights, whether real or imaginary, can lead to bad feeling which festers and ruins trust and mutual respect.

This itself may result in depression, and brooding has a habit of erupting in anxiety-ridden arguments, which cannot be good for any relationship. It is often better to say what you feel when you feel it, and then take positive steps to work out mutually satisfying solutions.

Oddly enough, it is known that fewer couples suffer from depression than single, separated, divorced or widowed people. Although relationships with other people are a chief cause of anxiety and depression, having someone you love available for some sympathy and reassurance obviously helps. And good, strong, honest, loving relationship can do a lot to help you avoid these problems.

Coping with bereavement

Of course, one thing people in our society are very reluctant to talk about is death. I have already said that the death of someone close to you is a natural and normal cause of depression, but let's look at it a little more closely.

When someone dies, whether it is the result of a long illness or something sudden like an accident, your first feeling might be one of shock. Recently bereaved people can react in many ways, often depending on their characters; it is very common – obviously enough – to feel unhappy and miserable, to cry and even think that life is not worth living any more.

Other common feelings – which people are not encouraged to talk about, and which therefore often make them feel guilty – are anger and resentment at being 'left', and guilt for all the things which you might regret having said or done to the person who has died. It is also usual to start thinking and worrying about the fragility of your own life when someone close to you dies. You begin to realize that you too will die one day – and that, of course, can be very saddening.

As I have already said, it is important to remember that all this is normal and that it needs expression. Early on after a bereavement, you might not feel like talking about the person who has died. You might prefer to live in the past a little, think of the good things you have lost, and concentrate on something you value by working through your memories – this does help.

There will almost certainly come a time when you want to pick up the threads of your life once more and that is the time when you need someone to talk to, someone to help you find your feet. Again, the guidelines I have given further on in this chapter for coping with stress will help. But remember that grief is natural, that it needs to be worked through and not repressed. Grief that is denied will fester and may lead to a serious depression. Letting the grief of bereavement come out is a great help to getting over it. I shall be giving advice about the use of drugs during this difficult time in Chapter 5.

Coping with changing responsibilities

I have already talked about the part that loss can play in depression, and I have also spoken of grief as the natural result of a loss. Some experts believe that loss is the essential problem in depression, and certainly loss and grief will affect all of us as we grow older in ways you might not expect.

Adolescence   For example, the depression many adolescents go through is often the result of losing the security of childhood. At puberty, children begin to see that they will eventually have to go out into the world, stand on their own feet, look after themselves. All this can be daunting and in this sense it is quite natural to 'grieve' over what you leave behind – the known, the safe, the comfortable – as you launch out into a new role in life with which you are as yet unfamiliar. This uncertainty about future status can in itself lead to anxiety.

Marriage and parenthood   The same is true of marriage and parenthood. Marriage – however much you love your partner and want to marry – can mean the end of being single and all the freedom that entails. Parenthood is a major change in your life, involving you in new responsibilities, great demands on your time, energy and material resources, all of which can make you feel depressed. Again, it is a question of 'losing' a familiar status and launching into a new area of life which is unknown and fraught with difficulties and anxieties.

Retirement also involves a loss of status for many people. You might have worked all your life, and enjoy your work relationships. Getting up, going to the office and coming home five days a week, forty-eight weeks a year, gives your life a structure; a job well done gives satisfaction and a sense of personal worth. After retirement all these things are missing, and many people find that they simply do not know what to do with their lives any more. They miss work, and so grieve – and become depressed.

Difficulties like these can be solved by two things: preparation and open acknowledgment. Our society is bad at exploring and recognizing these transitional events in life. That is why adolescents so often feel misunderstood, and parents are reluctant to talk about the negative feelings they might have towards their children or their situation. People who are about to retire are often more likely to be told they are lucky and that they will have a wonderful time with all that 'freedom' than that they may feel depressed.

More attention is being paid to these problems, and it would help us all to understand that there can be bad as well as good sides to every change in status, however positive it might seem. This would probably make it easier for people to acknowledge their feelings if they find themselves depressed in these situations, and getting these feelings off their chests would be a good start in overcoming them. The guidelines that follow will also help.

PRACTICAL MEASURES

By now we are in a position to put together some guidelines on coping with the problems of everyday life. One thing we have seen is that anxiety and depression have physical effects as well as emotional ones. Taking steps to control these will help you regain some energy and will-power to deal with your problems more effectively.

Adapting your life-style
Take a break This might help you to relax, get things in perspective, or come to terms with your problems.

Keep occupied Take up a hobby (painting, pottery, chess, drama, photography, for instance) or evening classes – anything that will motivate you and help to take your mind off your problems.

Try to get a little enjoyment into your life   It is important to look actively for pleasurable experiences. Try having an evening out, reading a good book, listening to a record which you enjoy, going shopping and buying yourself something just for the fun of it. Do not dwell on the things which make you feel anxious or might add to your depression – make a conscious effort to do whatever you like doing.

Take action   Consider your problems one by one, and if you can think of any form of positive action which will help – however minor – take it. Try to solve the easiest problems first. Success breeds success – if you can overcome one problem it will give you the strength and confidence to tackle more. An added incentive would be to reward yourself for every goal achieved – perhaps with one of the suggestions made in the previous paragraph.

Talk it over   Support from your family and friends is vital. If you do not find someone who is sympathetic, keep looking until you do. It is important for you to get things off your chest.

Take some exercise   Physical activity is an excellent way of coping with depression and anxiety, whether it is a gentle walk to help you mull things over, a regular jog round the park, or a furious game of squash which lets you take out all your frustrations. It will help to clear your head and make you feel better in yourself. Physical well-being is an essential foundation for mental well-being, and keeping fit plays an important part in helping you to maintain your self-confidence and self-esteem. Exercise should even help you get a better night's sleep (see page 34).

More and more people are becoming health conscious and are taking up exercise and sports. I am all in favour of this. A reasonable degree of fitness can be achieved at any age, but you need to be careful, especially if you have not exercised before, or for a long time. To avoid damage to your body, you should take up your new activities gradually.

For example, you should only jog a short distance to start with, and stop as soon as you feel breathless or pain in any part of your body. When you are used to jogging a short way then you can try increasing the distance a little at a time. If you are in any doubt, consult your family doctor. A good all-round exercise with little likelihood of doing damage is swimming. This is an activity which it is easy to take up gradually, too.

Eat regularly   When you are feeling down, you may lose your appetite. If you find you can't manage a proper meal, at least try to eat wholesome snacks through the day. These will give you the energy you need to take some of the other steps recommended above.

Try to relax   Relaxation is vital, especially in our modern, stress-filled world. If you can, set aside some time every day to relax a little and unwind. Try to empty your mind and forget your troubles – it will make you feel better. In the following section I have given some practical suggestions on how to relax.

How to relieve tension
We have seen that tension is one of the major symptoms of anxiety, and it can be part of depression, too. There are several well-tried, easy-to-follow techniques that you can use to relieve tension – and therefore lower the level of adrenaline (epinephrine) in your body, which in turn lessens the physical symptoms, such as faster heartbeat and breathing, and excessive sweating. One of the great advantages of these methods is that they are entirely under your control.

Relaxation   One of the simplest and most thoroughly proven methods is muscle relaxation. This involves the recognition of unnecessary muscle tension, learning how to release it, and then using these techniques in everyday living situations. A good way to start is to tense different groups of muscles and then relax them, in a logical sequence (see illustrations on pages 30–2). However, some anxious people find that the strong contracting of the muscles makes them feel more on edge, so it is best to drop the tensing part of the exercise once you have got the feel of exactly where the muscles are that need to be relaxed. When you are able to release all the tension, you will feel pleasantly calm and rested.

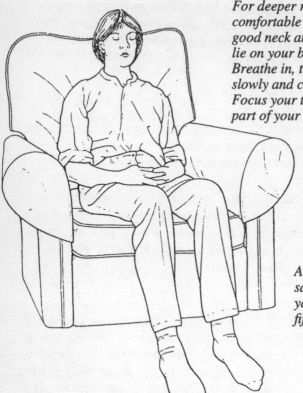

For deeper relaxation choose a comfortable chair or sofa with good neck and back support, or lie on your back on the floor. Breathe in, then breathe out slowly and close your eyes. Focus your thoughts on each part of your body in turn.

Always keep to the same order and give yourself at least fifteen minutes.

1. *Relax ankles and legs, rolling outwards.*
2. *Let arms and hands feel heavy and limp.*
3. *Relax your back when it's fully supported.*
4. *Drop and relax shoulders.*
5. *Let neck feel easy and relaxed.*
6. *Relax face with lips and cheeks soft, jaw loose and forehead smooth.*
7. *Let breathing become gentle, slow and even.*

After relaxing you can go on to any of the quieting techniques you find useful (see pages 32–3).

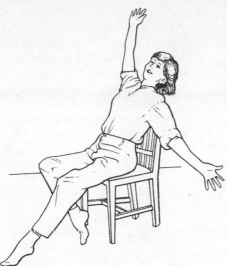

Learning to recognize tension and relaxation *Once you have tried these exercises a few times, there will be no need to tighten up the muscles before you relax.*

Have a good stretch. Then relax as you breathe out.

Ankles and legs *Straighten out one leg and bend up your foot at the ankle. Hold thigh tight and recognize the hardness and tension with your hand. Then relax and feel the difference. Repeat with other leg.*

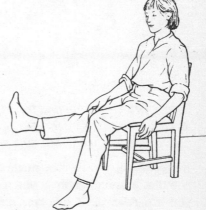

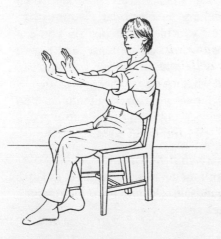

Hands and arms *Stretch out and tighten your fingers and arms. Be aware of the feeling of tension, then relax so that your hands and arms feel heavy and floppy.*

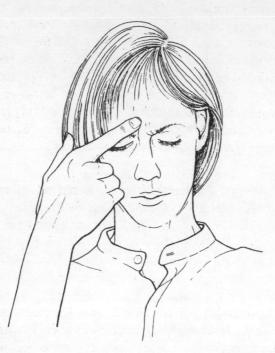

Face   *Grit your teeth and frown. Feel the ridge of tension in your forehead with your finger. Relax, letting your jaw drop a little and notice your forehead becoming smooth.*

Biofeedback   This is a method which is becoming increasingly popular. It actually allows you to hear when you are tense and when you are relaxed. It involves attaching an electrical instrument to fingers or groups of muscles. After you have switched on you can listen to the rising pitch of the buzz when you are tense, and how it lowers to almost nothing when you are relaxed. In this way you can discover what makes you tense and what makes you become calmer. It is a way of learning to have control over your anxiety feelings. You will find that with repeated experience you will be able to manage without the instrument. See Chapter 11 for useful addresses.

Quieting techniques   There are a number of methods that involve simple mental exercises which can quieten down a restless, anxious mind. They all benefit by learning muscle relaxation first (see above). The best known of these techniques are:

1. **Autogenic training**   This method originated in Germany but is now being taught under medical supervision in many Western countries. Relaxation is usually taught first, followed by a series of mental exercises. These involve focusing on sensations of warmth and heaviness in your limbs, calm easy breathing, calm heartbeat, cooling of the forehead. An example of this is allowing yourself to be affected by the phrase 'My arm is heavy and warm' or 'My breathing is calm and even.' Some autogenic training organizations are listed in Chapter 11.

2. **Meditation**   This has ancient origins and many forms are used today. Meditation involves focusing your mind effortlessly on a neutral subject such as a word or meaningless sound (known as a 'mantra'), the rhythm of your breathing, a sentence, a prayer or a visual image. You let your mind be filled with these, and emptied of your problems. As we have already seen, taking your attention off your troubles is important in coping with anxiety and depression. Once you have acquired the technique, you can practise it a few times daily, especially when you feel tense.

Many people learn to meditate in conjunction with yoga – special physical exercises involving precise control of posture and breathing. The beneficial effects of these methods, combined with biofeedback (see opposite), are well established by research.

Controlling your breathing   The way you breathe is very closely related to how you feel. When you are anxious or upset your breathing becomes irregular, or gasping, and takes place in the upper part of your chest. In contrast, when you are relaxed your breathing is slow, even, and mainly in the lower part of your chest, with a pause at the end of the out-breath.

Some people, especially when they are anxious, habitually overbreathe without realizing it, sometimes upsetting the chemical balance between oxygen and carbon dioxide in the blood. This can make you feel dizzy and faint and makes anxiety feelings even worse.

You can help yourself through a difficult situation with the following emergency technique. As soon as you feel that you are getting anxious or upset, say to yourself: 'Stop it!' (that means stop getting so worked up). Then breathe in, gently, and not too deeply. Breathe out slowly and as you do so deliberately let your shoulders drop, and then relax your hands. Pause for a moment and say to yourself 'Relax', or if you prefer, 'Calm'.

Repeat this once or twice more, thinking just about your breathing out and relaxing. You can do this anywhere without anyone noticing, and you will find that it lowers the tension enough to quieten the turmoil before it gets out of hand. It is a simple, but extremely effective self-help method of coping with an anxiety attack, that is worth practising straight away so that you are well prepared for the next time you need it.

Massage Some people find massage – performed either by themselves, their partners or by a professional masseur – very relaxing indeed. Again, it is a question of relieving the physical symptoms of anxiety and tension (see page 36).

If you want to know more about coping with stress and tension, you can do no better than read *Stress and Relaxation* by Jane Madders.

What can you do about insomnia?
Sleeping difficulties are very common – around 15 per cent of patients seeing their family doctor report trouble sleeping – and insomnia plays a part in both anxiety and depression. We all know how much more difficult it is to get to grips with anything in life when we are feeling drained and bad tempered through lack of sleep. And difficulty with your sleep can itself aggravate your anxiety or depression. If you are tense and anxious, then not going to sleep might just be another source of worry. Worrying that you will not get enough sleep to enable you to cope with the day ahead will only make you less likely to get off to sleep in the first place. Furthermore, if you are depressed, a few restless nights might start you thinking that you have some sort of dreadful illness – and give you something else to be miserable about.

So it is important to realize that not going to sleep until the early hours of the morning is not going to do you serious mental or physical harm. Many people go through their whole lives with very little sleep and suffer few – if any – ill effects. What is important, though, is to feel happy with the amount of sleep you are getting, and of course if you find that you are drowsy in the day it might pay to sort out your sleeping habits. Here's a list of 'golden rules' for getting a good night's rest.

1. Try to stop thinking about your problems or doing anything taxing in the evening. The more you fuel your mind, the longer it will tick over during the night. You need calm, quiet relaxation. Many people find that reading is a good way to wind down.

2. Don't eat a heavy, indigestible meal shortly before you go to bed. But don't go to bed hungry – the pangs might keep you awake.

3. Make sure your bed is comfortable and your bedroom neither too warm nor too cold.

4. Smoking just before you go to sleep is doubly unwise. First, it can be a real fire risk; and second, nicotine is a stimulant which raises the blood pressure, increases the production of adrenaline (epinephrine), and may keep you awake.

5. Regular physical exercise during the day will make your sleep easier and more rewarding. Sex too may leave you sleepy, although some people find the stimulation makes them more aroused and wakeful than they were beforehand. Even if sex does help you get to sleep, it is not fair to your partner to treat love-making as merely a means to this end.

6. Going to bed at a regular time will help to give you the most refreshing sleep. Your body has a natural sleeping rhythm which suits you, and the more regular your sleeping habits, the better.

7. If you find you are not going to sleep and you are getting anxious about it, use some form of relaxation technique (see pages 30–2) to help yourself calm down and drop off.

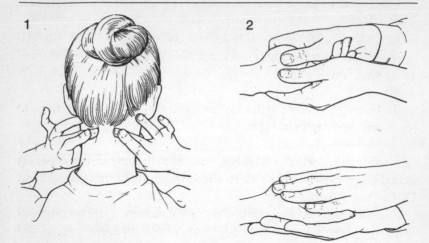

Massage *1. To relieve a tense aching neck, make circular, pressing movements with your fingertips around the base of your skull, then down each side of the spine.* *2. Rest your partner's hand on yours, then make circular pressing movements all over the palm with your thumb. Finish by stroking her hand between yours.* *3. Stroke slowly, gently and rhythmically with the whole of a relaxed hand across the forehead and to the opposite temple. Repeat the other way with the other hand. Finish by stroking upwards over the head and down the back of the neck.* *4. Roll firmly upwards with your thumbs (it must not feel uncomfortable). Then smooth your hands down each side of the neck.*

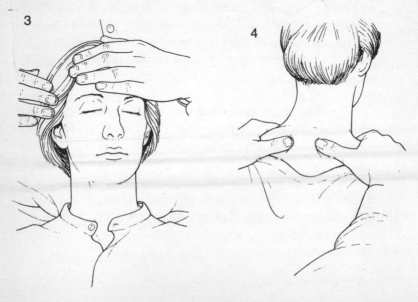

8. Try not to lie in bed tossing and turning; it will only make it harder to get to sleep. Find a totally comfortable position and stick to it if you can.

9. Getting up earlier in the morning will also make it easier to go to sleep promptly at night.

A useful book which will help if you are suffering from insomnia is called *Get a Better Night's Sleep* and is by Professor Ian Oswald and Dr Kirstine Adam.

But what happens if you take the positive action I have recommended in this chapter and your anxiety or depression doesn't go away? And what can you do when you feel depressed or anxious for no obvious reason? I shall be explaining in the next chapter how your family doctor can help you in these situations.

4
WHEN TO GO
TO YOUR DOCTOR

Anxiety and depression are very common, and there must be many people who are reluctant to go to their family doctors for help. It is easy to see why; people tend to think of doctors as 'body mechanics', experts in sorting out physical illnesses like coughs, stomach upsets or cuts and bruises.

If you have got a sore throat, you can go along to your doctor, and he will be able to tell you what is wrong. He might also be able to give you some medication to clear up the problem. On the other hand, a vague feeling of tension and unease, or a depression that you cannot shake off, might not seem so easy for your doctor to sort out.

However, it is important for you to go to your doctor if you cannot overcome your anxiety or depression with the self-help methods I described in the last chapter. First and foremost, your doctor can put your mind at rest simply by giving you a clean bill of health. He can see that you have blood tests to find out whether you have an overactive thyroid gland. He can give you a thorough medical examination to make sure there is nothing wrong with your heart, and arrange for you to have an electrocardiogram (ECG or EKG) and blood-pressure tests as proof that your heart and circulation are in good condition. Just knowing that you are physically healthy despite your fears could be a great relief in itself. Of course, if there is anything wrong, your family doctor will be able to give you treatment or refer you to a specialist to get the problem under control and cured.

Your doctor is not simply a 'body mechanic'. He is well aware that illness can sometimes be as much in the mind as in the body – or affect both together. In that same survey I conducted into people in Britain who go to their family doctors with emotional problems, I found that a doctor can expect to see on average one patient every day with anxiety or depression, or a mixture of the two. That means that your doctor probably has a lot of experience in dealing with this sort of emotional distress.

It is true that not all doctors are trained in dealing with problems of the mind, but most have the practical experience to know that many of the illnesses they see have more to do with anxiety or depression than physical causes. If you have a good relationship with your doctor, one of the best reasons for going to see him is that you feel he is someone you can talk things over with and who can help you. In Chapters 5 and 6 we shall also see that your doctor can give you direct help in the form of drugs, which can sometimes make all the difference in helping you to overcome your problem.

Remember too that he can put you in touch with specialists other than doctors, such as social workers or marriage guidance counsellors (see Chapter 11). Some people are lucky enough to have doctors who will even go further and talk to organizations or individuals who might be causing you distress, such as your employer. It is not always so – but look upon your doctor as your second line of defence, after your family and friends, and as the first major step in devising a strategy to beat your anxiety or depression.

WHEN TO SEEK HELP

You might know that it is time to seek help when one or more of the following things applies to you.

1. Your problems seem to be completely on top of you and there does not appear to be a way out.

2. Your whole life is being disturbed by anxiety and depression. If your relationships, your job or your health are suffering, then it is time to seek help.

3. Life seems unbearable, either because you are so fed up or because you know that whatever it is that makes you feel anxious is unavoidable.

4. You have lost the confidence – and the will – to carry on.

5. You have so many symptoms of anxiety and depression – like

trembling hands, excessive perspiration, palpitations, strange aches and pains (see Chapters 1 and 2) – that you are continually worried about the state of your health.

Don't hold back

Even though you feel a visit to your doctor might be helpful, you may still be reluctant to go. Doctors, hospitals and medicine can all provoke anxiety in even the calmest of people, having as they do connections in our minds with illness, pain and other unpleasant subjects. For someone who is anxious, there is the added worry of going to your doctor and talking about the things which make you feel that way. If you have not found much sympathy in those around you either, it might be frightening to go to this figure of authority – whom you might not know very well – and lay bare your soul.

If you have anxiety and depression which seem to have no real cause, you might also fear that you are going insane. As we have already seen, this is unlikely to be the case. Just because you go to your doctor with an emotional problem certainly does not mean that you will be dragged off to an institution against your will. This just does not happen.

If you are depressed you may tend to experience feelings of guilt and unworthiness. When you are feeling gloomy, pessimistic and not worth anybody's care and attention, it is easy to believe that you should not bother your doctor with your 'minor' troubles, and that there are many other people who need his help and time much more than you.

If you can, it is important to stop yourself from acting this way. Your doctor is there to help you. It is what he is trained for, and what he is paid to do, and if your problem is important to you, it will be important to him. That is not to say all doctors are perfect – but you have an excellent chance of getting sympathy, reassurance and help from your doctor in sorting out problems which are potentially very serious if left untreated.

When you might not realize that you need help

Another difficulty is that sometimes you may not realize that you are suffering from anxiety and depression. For example, a man who has palpitations, breathlessness and some vague aches and pains may go to his doctor worried that he is suffering from a heart condition.

If he doesn't admit to any other symptoms or personal worries, and if he conceals his insomnia and his feelings of panic, his doctor may think that his patient is only concerned about his heart. After telling him that physical examination shows his heart to be healthy, the doctor may think that this is the end of the matter.

Of course this has not really solved the problem of his patient's general state of anxiety. The man may have put all his anxiety down to fear of having a heart attack. His real difficulty could be that something in his life – or several things in combination, such as financial and marital problems – is making him feel anxious, and this anxiety is in turn producing the palpitations. The more he goes on having to put up with the palpitations, the more he worries, just increasing his state of anxiety in a vicious circle.

People with severe depression and anxiety often find it very hard to believe that they are suffering from anything other than a physical condition. The same man might go back to his doctor if the palpitations continue, and insist on another examination. If the doctor still finds nothing wrong, the man might demand a second opinion. It is known for people with anxiety and depression to go on demanding further examinations until finally a doctor or specialist manages to convince them that their condition might be emotional.

It is important to be aware that anxiety and depression can cloud your judgment. If you are depressed, for example, you might find yourself concentrating on your physical symptoms in a pessimistic way. Being told by your doctor that there is no real cause for your aches and pains or sleep problems except that you are depressed might not be a very welcome answer. One reason for this is that, as I have already said, people tend to associate all emotional ill-health – or ill-health of the mind in general – with psychiatrists, and therefore with insanity. I must repeat that having an emotional problem does *not* mean that you are going mad, so acknowledging it as such should hold no fears, and is an important first step on the road to recovery.

This difficulty in recognizing and accepting anxiety and depression holds important implications both for sufferers and for those who have a depressed or anxious friend or relative. For sufferers, it is vital to realize that something other than physical causes might be at the bottom of your unpleasant symptoms. You should try to keep an open mind on your doctor's advice. That is partly what this book is attempting to help you do. I am trying to make more people aware that anxiety and depression are the root causes of much suffering in our society. If you bear that in mind when you next visit your doctor, he might have a better chance of helping you.

If you are reading this book because you suspect that a friend or relative is suffering from the effects of anxiety or a depression which they do not recognize, then remember that they may react with shock or surprise if you say they might be suffering from one or other condition. They are more likely to say that all they need is help with a specific difficulty like lack of sleep, even though they might be very pessimistic about the chances of solving it. What they need is some gentle persuasion to get them along to the doctor – and some support in understanding that they are not imagining things, but simply have an emotional problem which their doctor can help to solve.

HELPING YOUR DOCTOR TO HELP YOU

The most important thing to remember about your doctor is that he is human. We tend to think that doctors have all the answers, and that all we have to do is to describe our symptoms and he will give us something to make us better. But your doctor is not telepathic; the only way he has of finding out what's wrong and doing something about it is to examine you and talk to you. If you hold something back from him, then you are not giving him a fair chance – and that means you are not helping yourself.

So it is important to tell your doctor everything that you think might be relevant to your case. That does not mean that you have to tell him your whole life story. Doctors are usually very busy, and yours may not be able to give you much time at your first appointment. If you help your doctor to understand your problem quickly, then he may be able to arrange a longer appointment with you later on.

You should also bear in mind that doctors, being human, often vary a great deal in their approach to anxiety and depression. They are increasingly being trained to recognize and deal with them, but even so, your doctor might not have had the appropriate training and experience. It is still worth seeing him. If you let him know that you feel you are anxious or depressed and need help, the chances are that he will be sympathetic and attempt to give you that help.

Getting the best from your doctor

With all this in mind, the following plan of action might help you to get the best from your doctor.

Your appointment   If your doctor has an appointment system, try to make an appointment on a day when he is not too busy. This might mean you have more time to explain your troubles, and that he is more receptive because he is under less pressure.

Keep to the point   Try not to be vague. Explain your symptoms as briefly and concisely as possible, and leave nothing important out. If you are frightened you have a heart condition because of palpitations you are not going to help yourself by not mentioning it.

Mention the causes   Tell him if you think that there is an obvious cause for your anxiety, your depression or your other symptoms. He may be able to help in very specific ways, perhaps by intervening on your behalf with the people or organizations (like your landlord, your employers and so on) who are making life difficult for you.

Take notes   If you think you will find it hard to talk to him, write it all down beforehand. Take a notebook and note down any relevant information or advice he gives you. If you think you will be really nervous, ask your doctor if you can bring a friend or relative along. Both these things will ensure you remember what happens and also that you do not get anything out of proportion.

Try not to expect instant solutions   Your doctor will help you, certainly, but many problems take a long time to solve. Try to think of going to your doctor as another important step on the road to recovery.

Remember that if your treatment is State-funded and you are not satisfied with your doctor's treatment or advice, you are entitled to ask him to refer you to another doctor for a second opinion. If you are paying for your own treatment or you have private medical insurance you can, of course, simply choose to go and see another doctor.

WHAT PSYCHOLOGICAL HELP CAN HE GIVE?

Once you have talked to your doctor, he will probably examine you physically. This is, as we have seen, to make sure that you are not suffering from an illness which could cause the same symptoms. If you are given a clean bill of health, then he may well diagnose 'depressive illness' or an 'anxiety state' and set about treating you himself.

In most countries family doctors themselves treat up to 90 per cent of the people who come to them suffering from anxiety or depression, and send less than one patient in ten to specialists for extra help. One reason for this is that your doctor is there and wants to help you – and he might well have the skill and experience to do so successfully. Another reason is that in most countries there are fewer psychiatrists than family doctors, and in those whose health services are State-funded you might have to wait several months for an appointment. Although it is more common in North America than in Britain or Australia for people to go straight to a specialist with anxiety or depression, most American sufferers will in fact be treated by their family doctor.

One other thing it is important to mention is that most people with emotional problems make a speedy recovery with their doctor's help and advice. That is what he will give you – advice and counselling, and above all, understanding. In the next two chapters we shall look at the drugs your doctor may give you. Here I shall concentrate on the psychological help he can offer.

Reassurance
One of the most comforting things that your doctor can give you is reassurance. Above all, he can reassure you that your physical symptoms can be overcome and that there is nothing seriously wrong with your body.

Reassurance about your mental anguish is not so easy to give or clear-cut. Suppose some loss or disappointment has really upset you. In this case it might not be a question of physical symptoms; it seems that your whole life has gone sour. You might react badly if anyone were to say to you, 'Don't worry, things aren't as bad as they seem.' It might sound even worse coming from your doctor. To begin with, you might feel that your doctor does not understand you or how bad things really are, otherwise he could not say such a thing. Anyway, how does *he* know? To you, things *are* as bad as they seem. You are the only person who can tell quite how bad they are – you might think – and that is why you are seeking help.

Attempts to reassure you, even when they are well-meaning, can often go wrong. It is important to remember that when you are suffering from mental pain – and that is what anxiety and depression are – you can be irritable and easily upset. Anxiety and depression can also make you feel very pessimistic, and extremely reluctant to accept help when it is offered. All the same, hearing reassurance from someone with the authority of a doctor can provide enormous relief, even just as a start in solving your troubles. For example, if you have been bereaved and have had feelings of resentment towards your loved one for 'leaving you', then your doctor's reassurance that this is quite a normal reaction could be a great encouragement.

Explanation
Another thing your doctor can do is to explain what is happening to you, remove the mystery and put your problems into the clear light of day. Anxiety and depression can be very frightening just because they are mysterious.

Again, you may find it hard to accept your doctor's explanation. If he tells you that your aching neck is not a sign of serious disease, but really just the result of your anxiety, you might be offended or frightened.

However, your doctor will be able to make it clear to you that although the root of your anxiety or depression is in the mind, your pain is not simply a 'figment of your imagination' with all that that implies in terms of 'wasting everybody's time' and being a 'hypochondriac'. He can explain how, when you are feeling anxious, various groups of muscles in your body, particularly those concerned with posture, can become tense for reasons we saw in Chapter 1, and that when the muscles are tense for hours – or even days – on end, they become painful. So the anxiety in your mind is translated into a physical feeling of tension, and eventually pain, in the neck.

It is quite easy to accept other examples of the way the mind and body work together – everyone knows about the pulse beating faster and the blood rushing to the cheeks when you see someone you love. Your doctor will try to help you understand that physical pains can come from mental causes – and that this does not mean that the pain only exists in your imagination.

Practical advice
You might not be satisfied merely with reassurance and explanation.

You might want some straight advice on how to solve your problems. Your doctor may well give you some advice eventually, and it will probably be good advice when it comes, but do not be surprised if he seems to be a little reluctant to come out with it right at the beginning. There are reasons for this.

Human beings are very complicated, intelligent creatures. When someone is anxious or depressed, it often seems to family and friends that there is an obvious solution. If it is that obvious, why doesn't the sufferer see it? It sometimes happens that there is a serious drawback to the 'obvious' solution which is not immediately apparent to an outsider. It might not even be all that clear to the person with the problem. Though he might be scarcely conscious why, he holds back from taking what could be a potentially disastrous step – even if on the face of it, it seems like the obvious way of tackling things.

For example, if it is your job that is making you anxious, then changing your job might seem like the obvious step to take. Leaving your job, though, might be the wrong thing to do in career terms. There might not be another job as good to go to. All sorts of problems can lie hidden in the easy answer.

So instead of simply saying: 'You had better change your job, then,' your doctor will probably say something like 'I expect you have given some thought to changing your job.' This will give you a chance to talk about the advantages and disadvantages of such a move, and thus help to clear things in your mind a little. It might even prompt you to come to a decision yourself without feeling obliged to accept anyone else's advice – and the fact that your decision is a positive act under your own control can do you nothing but good.

Doctors are also usually careful about giving advice for another reason. When you are upset or depressed, you can often be your own worst enemy. You might do something in desperation which would only serve to make things worse. We can usually accept or reject advice according to its merits; but when we are anxious or depressed our judgment can be clouded. We seem to lose part – or all – of the protective mechanism that prevents us from making mistakes most of the time. We might follow the wrong advice and make things worse.

Sympathy
Your doctor can also help by giving you sympathy. Of course, you do not have to have a medical degree to give someone sympathy. We

have seen that this, like the other things you can expect from your doctor, could come from friends or family too, but it is an important part of any doctor's 'bedside manner'.

Again, sympathy is fine if you are in the right mood to accept it. We cannot all always respond easily to friendly gestures, even under normal circumstances. The same reaction we saw with the doctor's explanations might get in the way of our accepting his sympathy. Anxiety and depression do make people uneasy in personal relationships, and often the slightest hint of impatience, a patronizing attitude or insincerity can drive them back into their shells.

Nevertheless, your doctor will try to be sympathetic, and it is important for you to realize that unless he understands what you need from him, he will not be able to give you help in the right way. Anyway, doctors are not saints, so although your doctor will probably see that you need to be drawn out a little, some doctors at some times might get it a bit wrong. This is no reason to give up on him immediately, though; if you follow my guidelines on page 43 on how to help him help you, you will have a better chance – and you could always try again another day.

A frequent cry from people with anxiety or depression is 'Nobody understands how I feel.' It is the sort of statement which, on the face of it, might make it difficult for someone else to show sympathy. If you are anxious or depressed, try to keep in mind that your doctor probably does understand. He has seen people with your sort of problem before, and may even have been anxious or depressed at some time himself. He has painful emotions himself, remember.

Encouragement

Depression and anxiety can partly be due to a lack of confidence. You might not have the willpower to take the steps which are necessary to overcome your difficulties, even when someone gives you the right advice. Despite knowing the right thing to do, you might continue to put up with a distressing situation just for lack of confidence to take the necessary – but potentially painful – steps.

It is at this stage that the encouragement your doctor can give you might well save the day. Once you have decided on a course of action it can be a great help to have someone you can go back to for more advice, more liberal doses of sympathy, understanding and reassurance.

'Go on, you can do it, you really can!' Words like these can work wonders from the right person at the right time. Again, your lack of self-confidence, your irritability and pessimism might all hamper you from accepting this encouragement. It is amazing, though, how even minor successes can help you overcome these negative feelings and move on to cope with other problems. Given properly over a period of time, encouragement from your doctor can make all the difference.

ONE WOMAN'S SUCCESS STORY

If we look at one particular woman's story, it will be easier to understand how your doctor can help. We will be looking at phobias (which are closely linked to anxiety) in detail further on, but her case worked out so well that it makes a good example here.

Jacqueline was a young married woman, with eighteen-month-old twins, when she went to see her doctor because of claustrophobia, or fear of enclosed spaces. She lived in an apartment block, and had had no psychological symptoms until she was six months pregnant. At that time she had had an unpleasant experience. She found herself trapped in the elevator in her block, and had remained there for twenty minutes while it continued to go up and down. She cried for three days afterwards, and for the remainder of her pregnancy walked up and down the eleven flights of stairs to and from her apartment.

By the time she visited her doctor, she had moved to a single-level house, although she was still very frightened of going in elevators. She was also afraid of going in buses and trains, and had to leave the door open when she was sitting in a parked car.

Her doctor was able to get her to talk about her situation. He felt that there must have been some added factor which was making the problem worse than it should be. In many cases like this, the fears gradually subside, but Jacqueline's were becoming more severe.

Jacqueline's doctor soon discovered some interesting facts about her background. She had known that her mother had always been nervous, but did not know that she also suffered from claustrophobia until she talked about her own phobia to her. Jacqueline's father was also not all that happy about heights, although, oddly enough, until his retirement he had been a crane driver. Yet whenever he visited his daughter in her eleventh-floor apartment he refused to look out of the window because he had a fear of high places.

The doctor also discovered that Jacqueline was not particularly happy with her domestic circumstances, either. This was mostly because of her husband's parents who lived nearby. Her mother-in-law came uninvited to visit her practically every day – and gave her opinion on what she was doing wrong in bringing up the twins. Her father-in-law inflicted himself on them almost every evening, and Jacqueline felt that he did things which were deliberately annoying, like waking up the children. She herself was shy and reserved, and found it difficult to express her feelings when she felt irritated.

So it was not surprising that Jacqueline had developed a severe anxiety state: there was a history of phobias in her family, she had been suffering from quite severe stress in her family life, and she had had an unpleasant 'triggering' experience.

Her doctor gave her a chance to talk about her anxieties to get them off her chest. He also encouraged her to take positive steps to remedy them, starting with some straightforward advice on how to deal with her husband's parents. In fact, she enlisted her husband's aid – and he told his mother not to come round so often. Jacqueline herself stopped trying to be so nice to her father-in-law, and generally began to feel much happier with life. Her initial successes helped her regain some confidence and she was able to deal successfully with other problems. Her claustrophobia quickly improved, and thanks partly to her own efforts and partly to her doctor's, she now leads a completely normal life, with no worries about going into enclosed spaces like elevators, cars or trains.

5
DRUGS FOR ANXIETY

I have already said that the best way of curing anxiety is to treat the cause. For example, if you are worried that you might lose your job, then grasping the nettle and talking the situation over with your boss might sort out the problem. If it does, and you are relieved of your worry, then your anxiety should clear up.

Of course, life is not always so straightforward. Going to see your employer may not produce any sort of result, good or bad, and you might continue to be anxious. We have seen that anxiety tends to breed more anxiety, so to break this vicious circle it may be necessary to provide you with some means of getting relief as soon as possible. If your anxiety is particularly distressing, and there is no practical way of altering your circumstances to cope with it, then your doctor may well prescribe some drugs to get you over the worst patch.

Before we go any further, I should point out that drugs usually have two names – a trade name, which starts with a capital letter, and a chemical, or generic name. Trade names often differ from country to country, so to avoid confusion in the text, I have used only those trade names which are common to most English-speaking Western countries.

FOUR TYPES OF DRUG

There are four main types of drug which your doctor might give you for anxiety.

1. Barbiturates
2. Major tranquillizers
3. Minor tranquillizers
4. Beta-blockers

Barbiturates
How they work   These drugs will both relax you by day and make you sleepy at night. To reduce anxiety and tension barbiturates are

prescribed in small doses. They were used very commonly for this purpose in the past, and are still given by doctors from time to time.

Barbiturates* and similar sedatives

Generic name	UK trade name
amylobarbitone* amobarbital* (US & Canada)	Amytal
amylobarbitone sodium* amobarbital sodium* (US & Canada)	Sodium Amytal
butobarbitone* butethal* (US & Canada)	Soneryl
chloral hydrate	Noctec
chlormethiazole clomethiazole (US)	Heminevrin
dichloralphenazone	Welldorm
meprobamate	Equanil
quinalbarbitone sodium* secobarbital sodium* (US & Canada)	Seconal Sodium

Side-effects   There are now recognized to be drawbacks in taking barbiturates. The main problem is that they are very powerful drugs. An overdose of barbiturates can lead to a coma and even death. If they have been prescribed for you, you must take great care in following your doctor's instructions on dosage. With fairly large doses during the day, you might fall asleep, or at the very least find yourself staggering, and suffering from slurred speech and double vision. If you take a barbiturate to sleep better, you may find that you feel drowsy and slowed-up for some of the following day.

In addition, taking large doses of barbiturates for a long time can lead to physical dependence, or addiction. If someone who is addicted to them stops taking them suddenly he can experience what are known as 'withdrawal symptoms'. These can range from shaking and feeling extremely anxious, to having fits and delirium tremens (the DTs), depending on how much of the drug has been taken for how long. That is why doctors are very careful in their use of barbiturates – for even though they may prove very effective in calming down someone with severe anxiety for a while, their long-term use is fraught with danger.

Because of these unwanted side-effects, around ten years ago doctors changed from prescribing barbiturates for anxiety to using tranquillizers (see the following sections). It is possible, though, that you are still on barbiturates. If you now feel you would like to switch to another type of drug, do ask your doctor. Those who have made this change generally experience few of the withdrawal symptoms – and then only to a mild degree – and often find they become less dependent on their medication.

Major tranquillizers

How they work These drugs are called 'major' because they are most often used to treat what specialists term 'major' mental illnesses – the severe disorders which lead to people having to spend some time in psychiatric units or hospitals. Many of these conditions can be relieved dramatically by using the major tranquillizers, although this lies outside the scope of this book.

More important, it is known that the major tranquillizers can relieve anxiety and tension in some people with less severe emotional problems. Around one person in ten being treated with anxiety-reducing drugs takes either major tranquillizers or barbiturates. The major tranquillizers help to lessen tension and promote relaxation, and also help to give you a good night's sleep. However, because they are quite powerful, if your doctor decides to prescribe one of these for you, he will give you a smaller dose than would be given to someone with a much more serious condition.

Side-effects If you are taking a major tranquillizer you may feel drowsy. The resemblance between them and barbiturates ends there, because in large doses their actions are quite different. Even after very large doses of major tranquillizers, you are very unlikely to go into a deep sleep or coma, and if you fall asleep you can still be roused quite easily.

There are also none of the other side-effects, like staggering, slurred speech or double vision. Interestingly, major tranquillizers never cause addiction either – so even if you take them for a fairly long time there are no physical withdrawal symptoms when you stop them.

Major tranquillizers

Generic name	UK trade name
benperidol	Anquil
chlorpromazine	Largactil
ZU clopenthixol	Clopixol
clozapine	Clozaril
droperidol	Droleptan
fluphenazine	Modecate; Moditen
flupenthixol flupentixol (US)	Depixol; Fluanxol
fluspirilene	Redeptin
haloperidol	Dozic; Haldol; Serenace
loxapin	Loxapac
methotrimeprazine	Nozinan
pericyazine periciazine (US)	Neulactil
perphenazine	Fentazin
pimozide	Orap
pipothiazine	Piportil Depot
prochlorperazine	Stemetil
promazine	Sparine
risperidone	Risperdal
sulpiride	Dolmatil; Sulpitil
thioridazine	Melleril
trifluoperazine	Stelazine

Minor tranquillizers

How they work   The pills which come under this heading are called 'minor' because they are used especially in the treatment of what doctors call 'minor emotional disorders', such as anxiety states. You might think that to describe such a painful problem as anxiety as 'minor' is a little insensitive. It is purely a technical term, and distinguishes anxiety, even when it is severe, from more major psychological illnesses – schizophrenia, for example. People with anxiety states, unlike people suffering from schizophrenia, do not usually see visions, hear nonexistent people talking about them, nor have strange and irrational beliefs. They remain in contact with reality, however painful that reality might be at times. ·

Four out of five people taking drugs to relieve their anxiety are prescribed minor tranquillizers, which include the range of drugs known as benzodiazepines. In this group you will find well-known drugs like flurazepam (Dalmane) that are often prescribed as sleeping pills. In fact – like barbiturates – all benzodiazepines can be prescribed as daytime tranquillizers or night-time sleeping pills.

The two main actions of this type of pill are the relief of anxiety and the relief of insomnia. They make you feel more relaxed and less fearful and they also reduce tension, both mental and physical. They act directly on tense muscles, and therefore help to relieve the aches and pains that might bother you if you are suffering from anxiety.

Side-effects   should not be a serious problem with the minor tranquillizers, but you should know about those that can occur. If you are taking one of these pills to help you sleep, then you may not feel any side-effects at all the next day, although if you take them to relieve your anxiety during the daytime you might feel drowsy. Some people don't like this feeling, while others who simply want relief from their anxiety welcome it and even feel comforted.

Because these pills relax the muscles, they might make you feel a little wobbly in the legs. Again, if the pills are helping to relieve the aching tension in the back of your neck, this might not worry you – but if you are taking the pills for another reason, this side-effect might be unwelcome. The minor tranquillizers might also affect your memory, making you slightly absent-minded, and some types can also take the edge off your self-control, leading you to behave impulsively at times or lose your temper.

Large doses of these pills over a long period can lead to staggering, slurred speech and double vision, especially if you are elderly.

People taking minor tranquillizers over a long period can become reliant upon them, although it is difficult to say whether this is a real physical addiction or a psychological dependence. In my experience it is uncommon to see anyone suffering from severe withdrawal symptoms when they stop taking the pills, although some people do feel very jumpy for a while afterwards. It is difficult to say whether this is really a withdrawal symptom or just a recurrence of the original problem of anxiety.

Benzodiazepines

Generic name	UK trade name
alprazolam	Xanax
bromazepam	Lexotan
chlordiazepoxide	Librium
clobazam	Frisium
clorazepate dipotassium	Tranxene
diazepam	Diazemuls; Stesolid; Valium
flunitrazepam	Rohypnol
flurazepam	Dalmane
ketazolam	Anxon
lorazepam	Ativan
loprazolam	Dormonoct
lormetazepam	Noctamid
nitrazepam	Mogadon
temazepam	Normison

How long you experience this feeling of being on edge depends on exactly what pills you have been taking, their dosage and how long you have been taking them. The first two weeks after stopping the pills are usually the worst, but the symptoms can last for up to six weeks if you have been on them for a period of years. Coming off the drug may require persistence, but your efforts *will* be rewarded in the end.

Beta-blockers
How they work   In recent years a type of drug which relieves two of the common symptoms of anxiety – palpitations and shakiness – has become available. The pills, called beta-blockers, are used mainly for treating high blood pressure. The drug blocks the action of the nerves (called 'beta' nerves) that make the heart beat faster and make the blood vessels contract. If the main symptoms of anxiety that bother you are a rapid, forceful heartbeat and shakiness, then your doctor may recommend beta-blockers. They have one big advantage – they have absolutely no habit-forming tendency at all.

Beta-blockers used to treat anxiety

Generic name	UK trade name
acebutolol	Sectral
atenolol	Tenormin
indoramin	Baratol
labetalol	Trandate
metoprolol	Betaloc; Lopresor
nadolol	Corgard
oxprenolol	Slow Trasicor; Trasicor
pindolol	Visken
propranolol	Inderal
sotalol	Beta-Cardone; Sotacor
tamolol	Betim; Blocadren

Side-effects Beta-blockers suppress many of the stimulating effects of adrenaline (epinephrine) on the body, which include raising the pulse and keeping your breathing passages (bronchi) wide open to let air in and out of your lungs. By slowing your pulse, beta-blockers may make you liable to faint. They may also cause wheezing, particularly in asthma sufferers. You should mention asthma to your doctor in any case, but especially if you are seeing him about your anxiety.

SHOULD YOU TAKE THESE DRUGS?

All this talk of side-effects might sound very off-putting, making the cure seem worse than the problem. You may think that it would be better to face the anxiety rather than take a risk of becoming addicted to a drug with dangerous side-effects.

There are several points to bear in mind here, though. The first is that your doctor is well aware of the side-effects of these drugs, as well as their benefits, and he is likely to have had a long experience in using them in the correct way to break anxiety's vicious circle.

Second, it is important to remember that no drug is a miracle cure for anxiety. Life's difficulties simply do not go away just because you take a drug that calms you down. A minor tranquillizer does not eradicate the cause of your anxiety immediately, in the way that an antibiotic might kill off an infection. There can be occasions when taking an anxiety-reducing drug makes all the difference, but usually they are something to take while you try to relieve your anxiety by other means, or wait for it to go away of its own accord with the passage of time. If you would really prefer to put up with the anxiety and all its symptoms rather than taking a pill, your doctor will probably give you every encouragement to do so.

Probably the easiest way of looking at this question is by thinking of how you might use a pain-relieving pill if you break your leg. You might take it to relieve the pain while you are in plaster, waiting for it to heal. The pill is not crucial to the actual healing process, but it does help to make life more bearable while nature takes its course.

Your doctor might also advise you to exercise your leg gradually once the plaster is off. In this case, taking a pain-relieving drug can also help. Doing exercises with its help may make a permanent difference to how well your leg heals.

In the same way, drugs can help when anxiety – or depression – threaten to disrupt your life. If you are in danger of avoiding facing up

to your difficulties because of anxiety, then a tranquillizer may ease
your worries enough to enable you to tackle them with a little more
zest. Not facing up to your troubles might allow them to get worse or
even multiply.

Drug treatment for anxiety is often best when your anxiety is likely
to be short-lived – if you are very nervous about a forthcoming
operation or exam, for example. Drugs can also offer you a temporary
breathing space which allows you to gather your energies and look at
your life a little more objectively with an eye to dealing with the things
that worry you.

There are some unfortunate people who simply cannot find a way
out of their problems. Life may be very difficult for them, and
although a doctor may not want to keep them on tranquillizers for a
long period, he may have no alternative, if only to give them enough
relief to keep going – in the hope that a solution can be found
eventually.

It is very hard to say precisely how long anyone should take pills to
cope with anxiety. We have seen that taking them for long periods may
sometimes lead to psychological dependence – and in some cases
physical addiction. So it is wise to be advised by your doctor, who will
probably use pills for as long as necessary to get your anxiety under
control – and no longer.

GETTING THE BEST FROM YOUR DRUG TREATMENT

Before I go on to look at the drugs which can be used to treat
depression, it is important to make some general points about using
drugs. These will apply equally to whatever type of drug you are
taking.

1. If you are certain about taking pills to relieve your anxiety, tell
   your doctor. Talk it over with him. If you feel you can carry on
   without them and try to solve your problems without their help,
   so much the better.

2. Don't be afraid to ask your doctor about the pills he prescribes
   for you. Ask about any possible side-effects, and what good they

are likely to do for you. Ask him how long he thinks you need to take them. Tell him about any other drugs you might be taking – harmless drugs can sometimes cause harmful side-effects when they interact with other drugs already in your system.

3. If you are pregnant, or even if you just think you might be, tell your doctor (see Chapter 8). Drugs can harm the developing baby, sometimes causing handicap, and doctors recommend that you should take as few pills as possible throughout pregnancy – and aim to take none at all in the first few weeks.

4. Report any unwelcome side-effects or new problems to your doctor as soon as possible. He might be able to change your pill or reduce your dose.

5. Always follow your doctor's instructions and the instructions that come with your pills. Never take more than the stated dose, never give your pills to anyone else, and always destroy any that remain once your treatment is over.

6. Make sure your pills are locked away and out of reach of any children. Never leave them lying around. Even a small dose can be harmful or even fatal to a small child, who might be tempted to think that a brightly coloured pill is a sweet or candy.

7. The danger of the pills you are taking causing drowsiness, double vision or too much muscle relaxation ('wobbly knees') means that you should not drive, handle dangerous machinery or do anything else that needs concentration and could cause harm.

8. If you are taking any drugs that make you drowsy, such as barbiturates or tranquillizers, or some of the antidepressants (see next chapter), it is advisable to be very cautious about drinking alcohol, as the combined effect of the drink and the pills can be overwhelming – and even dangerous if large quantities are consumed.

ALCOHOL

To end this chapter I want to look at one of the oldest drugs used to relieve tension – alcohol. There is no doubt about it, alcohol is a drug, and although it is a very common one it can also be harmful.

Alcohol certainly relieves anxiety. People often recommend a good stiff drink before a daunting interview or any other anxiety-provoking event as a way of giving you confidence. A lot of people enjoy a drink of beer, wine or spirits at the end of the day exactly because it relieves tension, making their cares and worries seem a little bit less distressing. For some people it is only after they have had a few drinks that they can really enjoy life.

However, alcohol causes the same sorts of problems as some of the drugs mentioned in this chapter. First, it is only a temporary solution. It might take your mind off your worries and help you get to sleep, but they are still going to be there when the effect of the alcohol wears off.

Second, a large amount of alcohol will make you sleep very deeply. A very large amount taken in one session can even lead to you falling into a coma, which could be lethal: the coma might become so deep that breathing stops. This is very rare, but alcohol does have similar side-effects to barbiturates. Someone who has had a bit too much to drink might end up staggering, with slurred speech and double vision.

Regular drinking of large amounts of alcohol can also lead to physical addiction – alcoholism. The more alcohol you take, the more alcohol you will need to carry on getting the same anxiety-relieving effect. It is a slippery path downward to addiction and on the way down your problems are likely to increase. Alcohol costs money, and taken in excess it can destroy careers, lives and families. Like any other drug addiction, breaking out of it can be very difficult, with painful withdrawal symptoms such as delirium tremens (the DTs).

So although alcohol taken in small quantities might do no harm, you must always be aware of its dangers and inadequacy as a way of helping you through your anxiety. It is also something which people who are depressed can turn to in hope of solace – as we shall see in the next chapter.

6
DRUGS
FOR DEPRESSION

TRADITIONAL 'REMEDIES'
Drowning your sorrows
The idea of taking drugs to relieve your feelings of being depressed is not a new one. Alcohol has been used for this purpose for centuries, and 'drowning your sorrows' is just as common a reaction to depression as having a stiff drink is for anxiety.

This doesn't mean to say alcohol is an effective solution. Sometimes it is not successful at all, and it might make you even more depressed and tearful than you are already. Of course, getting very drunk will blot out your depression – but it will blot out everything else, too, and when you come round again your troubles will not have disappeared. We have already seen that anxiety can be made worse by alcohol – and the same is true of depression. On a very simple level, waking up on the morning after the night before, you might be made even more miserable by your hangover. If this sets you reaching for the bottle again, you can get trapped in a vicious circle. Obviously, as with anxiety, alcohol is no answer for depression.

Coffee and tea
'Have a nice cup of coffee and you'll feel better' is something people often say to others who are feeling low-spirited. It is often an attempt to get the person to open up and start getting his problems off his chest. As we have seen, this 'coffee and sympathy' therapy can play a valuable part in dealing with mild depressions.

Chemically, too, drinks like coffee, tea and cocoa can all be beneficial, as they all contain natural stimulants such as caffeine. Caffeine can improve several of the symptoms of depression. It can make you more lively, improve your alertness and make you feel happier. In this way it can relieve lack of energy, poor concentration and the sadness or melancholy that go with depression.

Unwanted effects   The effects of tea and coffee may well wear off
before the depression does, and so depressed people often find that
they are drinking more tea or coffee while they are feeling low. Since
caffeine is a stimulant, large amounts of it can cause palpitations,
trembling, insomnia and other symptoms which sound like features of
anxiety. So you could find, for example, that a cup of tea in the middle
of the night when you cannot sleep might make you feel better
temporarily – but it might also keep you awake later on.

Remember too that these drinks are habit-forming. If you get used
to drinking lots of tea or coffee while you're depressed, it might be
difficult to cut down when you feel better. All the same, many people
establish a balance, and drink enough tea or coffee to make them feel
better without finding they need to resort to the large doses that cause
the symptoms.

PRESCRIBED DRUGS

If you skipped the last chapter because you don't suffer from anxiety,
please turn back and read the section headed 'Getting the best from
your drug treatment' on pages 58–9. The points I listed there all apply
to the drugs used for depression, and it is vital that you should follow
these guidelines, especially on telling your doctor about any other
drugs you are taking, side-effects, and safety. It is important to be very
careful when you are taking any drug – and your doctor needs your
help in making sure that the treatment he gives you is safe, as well as
effective.

Just as with anxiety, there are a number of drugs that your doctor
can give you to deal with depression. However, drug treatments for
depression are a little more complicated than those for anxiety, so we
will need to go into rather more detail than in the previous chapter.
First we will look at how some of the drugs used to treat anxiety itself
can help people who are depressed.

Tranquillizers

We have seen that anxiety and depression are often linked, and that if
you are depressed you may feel the physical symptoms of anxiety.
Indeed, these symptoms – and the anxiety that causes them – may be
the thing that is making you depressed.

In this case, your doctor might well prescribe one of the minor tranquillizers (see pages 54–5) to help you calm down enough to start coping with your depression. They will also help you get a better night's sleep, something which could be vital. Tranquillizers are often used by doctors to help people who are suffering from milder, reactive depressions after disappointing or upsetting events. In these circumstances they can be a valuable prop to help you get through a particularly difficult time.

Amphetamines

Amphetamines or, more popularly, pep pills are stimulating drugs, which were used for the first time on a large scale during the Second World War to help aircraft crew stay awake during long missions.

Side-effects Until the 1950s they were also used by doctors to treat depression. They were, however, something of a blockbuster solution. Like caffeine, they make you more alert, more lively and happier. The problem is that they also produce insomnia, palpitations and trembling. They can be very powerful, too, making you talk incessantly, laugh at anything, move around a lot and even stay up all night.

They can also be addictive, and you need to take larger and larger doses to get the same effect. In excessive doses they have been known to cause mental illness. Their beneficial effects are short-lived, and as with alcohol, they might relieve your depression for a while, but are likely to leave you feeling worse the next day. So all in all, they were not a very effective treatment for depression. Doctors do not use them for this purpose any more, and it is important for you to realize that even if you could get hold of some pep pills they would probably do more harm than good.

Tricyclic antidepressants

How they work Much more useful are the drugs known as antidepressants. These were first used to treat depression in the 1950s, and the widest used are called 'tricyclic' antidepressants, because there are three rings in their molecular structure.

Unlike pep pills, these drugs appear genuinely to work on depression alone. In other words, if you take them when you are not depressed, you would not feel anything at all. They benefit only those who are suffering from depression already, and as a rule help them to get back to normal rather than to feel 'high'.

These tricyclic antidepressants are still the most commonly used drugs for the treatment of depression, so it is worthwhile looking closely at how they work. If your doctor prescribes them for you, the main thing to remember is that they will not start working for about ten days. If you are feeling depressed and apathetic it is easy to think that the pills are not working and give up before the first signs of improvement occur. So you need the commitment to stay on them long enough to give them a chance.

You might find that your sleep improves at first, or perhaps your appetite. Gradually your energy will return, and the future will not seem so gloomy. Often the most important effect is that your confidence comes back, so that you begin to feel able to make decisions again.

This improvement all takes place over a few weeks. Although it varies from person to person, most people will feel a lot better after six weeks on antidepressants, and will begin to believe that they will get over their depression after all. That in itself is a major breakthrough.

Side-effects The most common ones are a dry mouth, blurred vision and constipation. This is especially irritating if these symptoms are already part of your depression, as a dry mouth and constipation often are.

Another problem is that although the benefit of the pills can take several weeks to appear, the side-effects can come on in the first few days.

Tricyclic antidepressants

Generic name	UK trade name
amitriptyline	Lentizol; Tryptizol
clomipramine	Anafranil
desipramine	Pertofran
dothiepin	Prothiaden
doxepin	Sinequan

imipramine	Tofranil
lofepramine	Gamanil
nortriptyline	Allegron
protriptyline	Concordin
trimipramine	Surmontil

Some types of antidepressant pills have a tendency to produce insomnia as a side-effect, too – another common symptom of depression. It is more usual, though, for antidepressants to make you feel drowsy rather than wakeful. This drowsiness can be dangerous if you insist on driving or using complicated machinery, and it can also affect your ability to do your job properly. This could in turn make you feel more anxious and depressed.

However, it is not always necessary to take the pills during the day, as is usually recommended. With most types you can take a whole day's supply at bedtime, and use the drowsiness to advantage in fighting insomnia. By morning, the side-effect of drowsiness has often worn off.

If you experience side-effects it might mean that the dose you are taking is too high. How much of the antidepressant any individual needs to deal with his own particular depression varies enormously from person to person, with some people needing a dose ten times larger than someone else. A dose that causes side-effects in one person might cause none in someone else. How large a dose you need depends on you, and your doctor relies on you to tell him what effect the pills have on you – so do let him know!

Getting the dose right does depend on how you feel about the side-effects, too. If they are mild, you might prefer to keep on with the same dose to try and get the quickest improvement possible. If they are stronger you might want them reduced, even though taking a lower dose will mean that it will be longer before you feel better.

MAOIs

How they work   Other types of antidepressant drugs have also been developed since the 1950s. One type which now accounts for around 15 per cent of all drugs prescribed for depression is called a monoamine oxidase inhibitor. Even doctors baulk at using such a mouthful of words, and they are most commonly called MAOIs for short.

The effect of these drugs on depression was discovered when they were given to people suffering from tuberculosis (TB). Their original purpose was to kill the germ that causes this illness, but doctors soon found that it made depressed people – who were still very ill with TB – feel more cheerful. Research showed that they were not feeling happier simply because they thought that now the germs were being dealt with they would get better; the drugs themselves had a direct effect on their depression. Further tests revealed that MAOIs were indeed effective in treating depression, and there are now many different antidepressant drugs which come from this group.

Although chemically they are quite different from the tricyclic antidepressants described previously, in some respects their action is very similar. If you are given an MAOI, you are not likely to notice any improvement for the first ten days or so, just as with the tricyclics.

MAOIs

Generic name	UK trade name
isocarboxazid	Marplan
phenelzine	Nardil
tranylcypromine	Parnate

Side-effects However, some types of MAOI combine their anti-depressant effects with others which are like those of pep pills. They are likely to give you an extra boost, and they can be habit-forming. They can also cause dizziness and swollen ankles.

Another drawback with some MAOIs is that they can interact dangerously with other substances in your system. What happens is that they interfere with the process by which monoamines (chemicals in many of the common foods we eat) are broken down in your body. These accumulate in the bloodstream causing the blood pressure to rise, leading in turn to severe headaches, breathlessness and even, very rarely, burst blood vessels in the brain. The latter effects can be very serious indeed, causing a stroke or even death.

That is why your doctor will probably give you a long list of foods and drinks to be avoided while you are on MAOIs. The following are probably the most common.

Foods to avoid on MAOIs
- Cheese
- Yeast
- Beef and vegetable extracts
- Beans
- Pickled herrings
- Alcohol

You may well be given a card by your doctor with a full list of banned items. You should follow this rigorously, and always tell your doctor as soon as possible if you ever get any of the symptoms mentioned above while you are taking MAOIs. If you are ever treated by another doctor make sure that you let him know you are taking MAOIs. Finally, bear in mind that it is not advisable to have any type of anaesthetic – local or general – while taking these drugs. This includes dental anaesthetics, so do tell your dentist about your medication. You should also consult the pharmacist before buying over-the-counter medicines.

HOW LONG DOES IT TAKE TO FEEL BETTER WITH ANTIDEPRESSANTS?

To see how long it takes before you can expect to overcome your depression with antidepressant drugs, let us look at the case of a woman who has been depressed – for no apparent reason – for about a year. She probably goes to her doctor not really expecting much from him. In her pessimism and despair she does not believe that she is capable of being helped by anybody or anything.

He prescribes tricyclic antidepressants for her, and within a couple of weeks she is surprised to feel a slight improvement. She would like to think that the pills are really beginning to help her to get better, but she fears that it is just one of the temporary episodes which she has had from time to time when she has felt better for a while, only to get worse a few days later.

This time, though, she continues to improve. After six weeks she is almost back to normal. A few weeks later, and all traces of her depression have gone. She is back to her old self, grateful for the energy and confidence that have returned in full.

Antidepressant drugs are quite different from tranquillizers. It is common for anxious people to feel less tense within an hour or so of taking a tranquillizer – with antidepressants it is more a question of weeks. It is therefore necessary to take antidepressant drugs as a course of treatment. That means you will be taking them for a long period, regularly, day after day. If you stop them too soon, you may have a relapse.

Unfortunately there is no magic way of knowing how long you should take the antidepressants. Doctors have to rely on their experience and judgment, and yours will take into account factors like how long your depression has lasted, how severe it is, and how long it took to respond to treatment. In general, even where the depression had only lasted for a short time, was fairly mild and had responded quickly, the doctor will still recommend that you continue on the same dose for a full month after recovery. Where the depression has been more severe, he may well recommend that you stay on the pills for six months or even a year.

Your doctor will also probably take into account several other factors. If you do not like taking pills and are keen to come off them, he will stop them earlier, rather than later. On the other hand, if you would rather be safe than sorry, he may postpone the end of the drug treatment. You can probably work out with your doctor the best arrangement. Perhaps the right occasion to stop them would be a time when most things are going well in your life, and you feel you would be able to cope without the pills.

AVOIDING A RELAPSE

A relapse can happen if you stop taking the pills too quickly. Take the case I described previously of the woman who was depressed. Perhaps after six or eight weeks she feels much better, and thinks that now her problems are over it is time to stop taking the pills. She might be afraid of becoming dependent on them.

For ten days she feels fine. Then gradually, her symptoms of depression return, one by one and, within five or six weeks, she is just as depressed as she ever was. As we have seen, feeling depressed can make you feel very pessimistic. It can also distort your memory. People who are severely depressed tend to remember only the bad things about the past, and not the good things.

After a relapse like this it is sometimes very hard to persuade someone to go back on the antidepressants. She might say that they gave her a dry mouth and constipation. She might be very reluctant indeed to take the pills again, saying they did not do her much good. Even if she does agree to go back on them they might take longer to lift the depression the second time around.

That is why doctors are often reluctant to end the course of pills suddenly. They usually reduce the dose gradually. In this way, if you seem to be getting depressed again, he can put the dose back up to the maximum level that is best for you without any serious harm being done. If you are taking three pills a day, you might go down to two, then one, and then stop them altogether a week later. In more serious cases, the reduction can be even more gradual.

HOW EFFECTIVE ARE DRUGS?

It is difficult to say just how effective drugs are for depression. They are certainly one of the commonest forms of treatment, with literally millions of people taking them all over the world.

One reason why it is difficult to judge their effectiveness is that most of us are liable to a certain amount of suggestion, and if your doctor tells you that you will get well, then the chances are you will – whatever treatment he gives you.

Specialists often call anxiety and depression 'self-limiting' conditions. That is, they are likely to clear up by themselves eventually, even without any treatment. That is true, at any rate, of milder anxiety and depression. So if you go to your doctor and come away with a prescription for some pills and your doctor's assurance that they will help you get better, just the fact that you have done something positive and that someone is helping you might make all the difference. In this situation, you will probably have to go back from time to time to report on how you are getting on. This in itself gives you a chance to talk over your progress – and your troubles.

There is no doubt, though, that most people are helped directly by antidepressants. Some experts believe that those who are most likely to benefit are people with endogenous depressions – that is, those which 'come out of the blue', which no apparent cause – and that people who are depressed because of some upsetting event (reactive depressions) will fare less well on them. Some doctors also believe that they can tell precisely which sort of drug is suitable for which sort of depression. For example, if they decide someone is suffering from a certain type of depressive illness, they will give them MAOIs right from the start.

I am still unconvinced about this, though. It is true that people with endogenous depressions do better on antidepressants, but there are usually far more people with reactive depressions than endogenous ones. In their cases, antidepressants or tranquillizers often give them useful relief from their symptoms so that they can get on with the real business of solving their problems. Coming to terms with their feelings, making a new adjustment to their lives and their disappointments might be the best long-term answer.

For bereavement
In this context it is important to talk about grief. We have already seen that bereavement is a common cause of depression, and using drugs in the long term to help a bereaved person feel better may only make their grief worse by prolonging it. You need to grieve when you lose someone you love. You need to work through your feelings of anger, guilt and loss. Of course, these might be accompanied by unpleasant symptoms such as insomnia, which can be alleviated by drugs during the first few critical days. But if tranquillizers or antidepressants are used over a long period of time to help you feel better, you will still have to work through your grief later on when the drugs are stopped. If you do not, your grief could turn into a long-term depression. Oddly enough, drug treatments might be a help at that stage – when the depression has become out of proportion.

NEW DRUGS

The idea of picking a particular drug to deal with a particular type of depression is, of course, a very attractive one, which has recently received fresh encouragement. For a long time the choice of drugs has been between tricyclics and MAOIs; but in the last few years some drugs which do not fall into either group have been discovered, and these are sometimes called 'novel' antidepressants. Around one person in four taking medication for depression is now prescribed a novel antidepressant.

We saw that tricyclics have several side-effects, like blurred vision, dry mouth and constipation. Although none of the novel antidepressants of which I am aware is completely free of side-effects, there are some which are free of the ones I have mentioned in this chapter. More research is currently being conducted into these drugs, and I believe that in the foreseeable future we will be able to divide up depressive illnesses more certainly into those which do well on certain drugs, and those which do not.

Novel antidepressants

Generic name	UK trade name
amoxapine	Asendis
citalopram	Cipramil
fluoxetine	Prozac
flupenthixol	Fluanxol
fluvoxamine	Faverin
lithium	Camcolit; Liskonum; Priadel
l-tryptophan	Opitmax
maprotiline	Ludiomil
mianserin	Bolvidon; Norval
moclobemide	Manerix
nefazodone	Dutonin
paroxetine	Seroxat
sertraline	Lustral
trazodone	Molipaxin
venlafaxine	Efexor
viloxazine	Vivalan

PLAN OF ACTION

So in summary, when you visit your doctor with depression, his plan of action is likely to be as follows.

1. He will carry out a physical examination to rule out any illness which might have caused your depression.

2. He will try to find out from you what the cause or causes of your depression are, and may give you some practical advice. He will also probably offer you sympathy, understanding, encouragement and reassurance, as well as some explanation of depression and its effects.

3. If you are suffering from the symptoms of anxiety as well as depression, he may offer you tranquillizers. These may also be effective in dealing with some of the physical symptoms of depression, like insomnia.

4. He may offer you antidepressant drugs if your symptoms are giving you problems, or if it seems that there is no immediate practical solution that will help you feel better. These drugs may take some weeks to have any effect, and it is important to follow both your doctor's advice and the guidelines I have laid out on pages 58–9 on how to use prescribed drugs.

5. If your depression continues or the drugs do not work, he may switch you to another type of drug or change your dose.

6. Finally, he may refer you to a specialist for medical help which he cannot offer.

I shall be explaining what forms this specialist medical help takes in the next chapter.

7
SPECIALIST HELP

WHEN IS IT NEEDED?

It is encouraging that family doctors themselves are able to treat over 90 per cent of the people who go to them suffering from anxiety or depression. That still leaves a large number of people who cannot be helped by their usual doctors. Some of these people benefit from psychotherapy, and this is what I shall be looking at in this chapter. A word like psychotherapy might worry you, but it is just a general term for 'treatments of the mind' – and your family, friends and doctor may have been giving you just that, long before you get anywhere near a psychotherapist.

For example, in Chapter 4 we looked at the sort of psychological help your doctor can give you. This includes reassurance, explanation, advice, suggestion, sympathy and encouragement. This is, in fact, a specific type of treatment known as 'supportive psychotherapy'.

Psychotherapy is basically a talking treatment which may be given by a psychiatrist or a psychologist, and although sometimes drugs are used in conjunction with it, it is the talk and contact between you and your therapist which is important – and which produces results. There are many different types of psychotherapies, and the one which most people know about is psychoanalysis, a technique based on the work of Sigmund Freud. You are unlikely to come into contact with this form of treatment first, so although we will examine how this is done, we will look at the other major types of therapy, too. Before doing so, let's look at why your doctor might decide that you need this sort of help.

Why your doctor might recommend that you see a specialist
A difficult diagnosis Your doctor might not be absolutely sure about his diagnosis. He might think that your problems are not merely the result of a 'simple' anxiety state or depressive illness, but have a

more complicated cause or causes. If a delay in working out what was wrong would jeopardize successful treatment, then he will most certainly want to get a second opinion as soon as possible. After all, your family doctor specializes in not specializing – that is, he is trained to recognize a wide variety of problems and knows when you need more experienced help. He does the same when he seeks a specialist's help for a complicated physical problem.

Failure of treatment   If your doctor has been treating you himself and there has been no improvement in your condition over a period of time, he might also send you to a specialist. For example, he might have believed that your depression was mild and would respond to some advice and sympathy, with perhaps a short course of antidepressants. If there's no improvement – or if your depression gets worse – then he might decide you need some different help.

Danger signals   Your doctor will be keeping an eye out for danger signals from you, and if he sees these he will make sure you get specialist help as soon as possible. We have seen that people with anxiety and depression may be irritable and difficult to get on with. It is rare for them to act violently or aggressively towards others. What is not quite so rare is for them to have destructive feelings towards themselves. I shall be looking in Chapter 10 at how people with depression can sometimes feel suicidal. It is enough to say here that if your doctor detects in you any feelings like these he may want some extra help in dealing with them. Some doctors, though, are experienced enough to handle this sort of situation themselves.

A difficult relationship   Another reason your doctor might want you to see someone else for treatment is that your relationship with him has become difficult. The treatment of almost all illnesses, even physical ones like arthritis or influenza, goes much better if there is a good relationship between doctor and patient. Nowhere does this hold more true than in the treatment of anxiety and depression.

There are two points to be made here. One is that when you are anxious or depressed it is often hard to relate to other people. We have seen, in fact, that strains in your relationships with other people are among the most common causes of depression and anxiety. Under the stress of these feelings, it is easy to feel pessimistic about the chances of anyone – even your doctor – being able to understand or solve your difficulties.

The other point is that doctors are human too. You may just not get on with your doctor, just as you may not get on with your postman or a colleague at work. These things happen; it is all part of life. If the relationship between you and your doctor deteriorates to the point where you have no confidence in him at all, then it is unlikely that anything he says will help you. Doctors are generally alert for this possibility when they are treating patients with anxiety and depression, so when he feels that this is hindering your treatment, he will probably refer you to someone else who can help you more than he can himself.

Treatment he cannot give Finally, your doctor might recommend that you see a specialist because he believes you need treatment which he cannot give you. At the most basic level this might be a question of time. We saw that most people with anxiety or depression can be helped simply by having someone to talk to. Your doctor might realize that – and not have the time to give you the attention you need. Many family doctors could not even contemplate giving you one hour a week over an extended period to talk your problems over. I have said that you can expect some psychological and emotional support from your family doctor, but he will recognize when you have reached the stage when you need more than he can offer, whether it is a matter of the time he has or of his depth of experience.

Remember too that you do not have to wait for your doctor to refer you to a psychotherapist. You can seek one out yourself, although it would be wise to seek some advice from someone qualified before you make your final choice. The guide to the major types of therapy in the next section will help. This is because going to your own therapist will cost you money – and some treatments cost a lot more than others. Some, like psychoanalysis, may also last longer and be more demanding.

What sort of help is available also depends on where you live. There are fewer psychotherapists than there are doctors, especially in Britain and Australia. That is one reason why most people with anxiety and depression get their treatment from their family doctors – there are simply not enough psychotherapists to go round. You are also more likely to have access to psychotherapy in a city than in the country. In the United States and Canada, on the other hand, a psychotherapist is much easier to find – although again, this varies from area to area.

WHAT IS PSYCHOTHERAPY AND WHO GIVES IT?

All forms of psychotherapy involve a personal relationship and talk between the therapist and you. They are all methods of exploring possible causes of the problems in your mind, and helping you either to come to terms with them or to overcome them. The basic aim is for you to work through your problems and come up with a solution: either leading to a change in your attitude or a revelation of what it is that is really bothering you, which you can then do something about.

Before we look in detail at the types of therapy, it is important to draw a distinction between psychiatrists and other types of therapist.

A psychiatrist is a medical specialist. You cannot be called a psychiatrist at all unless you have qualified as a doctor. A psychiatrist takes his medical degree or diploma, and may then spend some time working as a family doctor or in a hospital, dealing with everything from cuts and bruises to major illnesses. From then on he will take a detailed training in the workings of and the treatment of disorders of the mind. He will be trained to recognize and deal with all sorts of emotional and mental problems, from the mildest of phobias to the most severe breakdowns. He is trained to use talking treatments – psychotherapy – but, because of his medical background, he is also able to prescribe drugs and use other treatments like electroconvulsive therapy (ECT), which I shall be describing in Chapter 10. He can recommend that you see a psychotherapist whose speciality is suited to your condition.

If he sticks to talking treatments and never prescribes drugs, a specialist doesn't need to have a medical degree to give someone psychotherapy. A psychologist is someone who has taken a diploma or degree in the workings of the mind. The sort of psychologist most sufferers from anxiety or depression are likely to come into contact with is called a clinical psychologist – in other words, someone who has a degree in psychology, and who has also been trained to recognize and deal with emotional disorders.

So what are the different types of therapy? Let's look at three major variations to start with.

SUPPORTIVE THERAPIES

Behaviour therapy

This is a form of therapy which is most often given by psychologists, although increasingly nurses in psychiatric units are being trained to use it. It is based on the work of the famous Russian scientist Ivan Petrovich Pavlov (1849–1936) whose experiments demonstrated that if a bell is rung every time a dog is given its food, eventually the dog will salivate as if in the presence of food simply when the bell is rung and no food is given. Salivating in the presence of food is a natural, or unconditioned, reflex. Salivating at the sound of a bell is a new reaction which the dog has learned – a conditioned reflex.

Behaviour therapy can be used to treat both anxiety and depression, although different techniques are employed for each condition.

For anxiety   The theory behind this kind of behaviour therapy is that the reaction of anxiety – phobias in particular – has been 'learned', and that it is possible for it to be 'unlearned'. The behaviour therapist will try to change your conditioned reflex to certain situations from being anxious, tense and afraid to being calm and relaxed. In the same way that Pavlov's dog learned by repeated training, you can learn automatically to relax whenever you begin to feel anxious.

First of all the therapist will want to find out from you what exactly it is that triggers off your feelings of anxiety. Then he or she will teach you a systematic technique for relaxing – probably similar to the one described in Chapter 3. Finally, you will be exposed to the trigger factor and be encouraged to relax whenever you start to feel anxiety coming on. Eventually this process should become a conditioned reflex action. This behavioural technique is often used to overcome phobias, and I shall be explaining two of its variations in detail in Chapter 9.

For depression   Behaviour therapy for depression is also based on learning a new set of responses. We have seen that when you are depressed you may feel too lethargic to take any practical steps towards recovery. The behaviour therapist will encourage you to behave in a positive way by setting you simple tasks – such as paying extra attention to your personal appearance, for instance – and will praise you when you carry them out. The aim is for you to 'relearn' the desire to get an enthusiastic reaction from the people around you. This should motivate you to take further positive steps, which in turn will lead to additional encouraging feedback – the very opposite of a vicious circle, and a simple, but often very effective way out of depression.

A similar treatment for depression, developed recently, is known as cognitive therapy. 'Cognition' is the technical term for an idea in the mind. Cognitive therapy helps you to get your mind off miserable, pessimistic ideas which only make you feel more desperate and which aggravate the underlying depressive emotions. Cognitive therapy is especially valuable since not only can it get you out of the depression that you are in, it can also help you to avoid depression in the future.

The behaviour therapies for anxiety and depression, although different, both help you to unlearn negative ways of responding to life's difficulties, and learn more positive 'conditioned' reflexes.

Assertion therapy
Being shy or unsure of yourself can lead to feelings of anxiety when you meet new challenges or come into contact with new individuals or groups of people. Assertion therapy, which is a specialized form of behaviour therapy, is aimed at helping you to achieve better ways of coping with such situations, and also to be basically more self-assertive. Paul's case illustrates well the methods used in assertion therapy and the results it often achieves.

Paul was a senior executive working in London for a major multinational industrial company. Although he was successful at his job, he was always very anxious when he was required to speak in front of more than five or six people, especially in a formal setting. Committees were a nightmare for him. One day he was told by the directors that they would like him to take the Chair at a conference in New York for 500 business people. The board of directors would also be present at the conference.

Not surprisingly, Paul experienced severe anxiety symptoms at the prospect. He found it difficult to sleep, could not concentrate, and was quick to lose his temper with his wife and children. Following an unsuccessful attempt to treat these symptoms with tranquillizers, his family doctor advised him to see a clinical psychologist for behaviour therapy. The psychologist's initial assessment revealed that Paul had a long-standing difficulty in asserting himself, underlying which was a fear of making a fool of himself in public. As there were only ten weeks to go before the conference, he was offered an intensive course of assertion therapy. This involved certain loosening-up procedures – such as shouting – leading on to acting the part of having heated arguments with the therapist. A rehearsal lecture was arranged at which Paul was encouraged to speak as loudly as he could and use elaborate gestures to fill the stage with his presence. The aim was that provided he was behaving in an overassertive way he would not feel anxious. Later on in his course, he would have to try to tone down his performance to make it acceptable for the conference. However, he was encouraged to err on the side of exaggeration on the day, as it was preferable that he should come across as overconfident, rather than quiet, timid and ill at ease.

Paul sent a telegram to his therapist on the evening of the event which read: 'The conference was great and so was I.' Not long afterwards he was offered a directorship of the company, largely – he says – as a result of his good showing at the conference. He now has no difficulty whatsoever in public speaking, although he is reluctant to give up his newly acquired flamboyant style; and, more important, is now much more confident in all his social relationships.

Social and marital therapy

We have already seen that unharmonious relationships with other people can be major causes of anxiety or depression. Social therapists work at making sufferers more at ease with other people. These therapists help sufferers to cope better with their relationships, and perhaps to see where they go wrong – enabling them to see when they are expecting too much or too little from other people.

In many ways marital therapy is similar to social therapy, although obviously it concentrates on the specific problems which may be disrupting a couple's relationship. The whole approach of marital therapy is based on the premise that anxiety or depression within a marriage is caused by something between the partners – it is not usually solely one or the other's fault, but something which both contribute to. Although married people tend to suffer less from depression than other groups, when one or both partners is severely depressed, the whole loving foundation of the relationship can be threatened, and the depression may also be very difficult to cure without outside help.

People tend to get into habits in their long-term relationships, and that is why many arguments between a couple may have different beginnings, but tend to follow the same general patterns. Marital therapists aim to help couples see what their underlying problems really are; whether it is one partner's parents interfering too much; or a major difference in attitude between partners either in expressing love and emotion towards each other, or in the upbringing of the children. Once the couple understand what lies at the root of their disharmony, action can then be taken to put their relationship back on to a good footing. The anxiety or depression caused by these stresses within a marriage may then be cured. Obviously this can take some time, and is not always totally effective. However, many marriages and relationships have been saved by marital therapists.

For the therapy to have a chance of succeeding, though, both partners must be prepared to go along to see the therapist – not necessarily together at first – and be equally prepared to accept his or her help and advice.

Group therapy

Like behaviour therapy, the final aim of group therapy is to help you change your behaviour as well as your feelings and overcome your anxiety or depression. It differs from behaviour therapy in that it is, as the name suggests, therapy for a group of people with one psychotherapist, rather than for just one individual. One advantage is that, with a group of eight or more sufferers at a time to one therapist, it is more economical. Its benefits, however, go deeper than that.

Group therapy can sometimes bring about changes which individual treatment cannot accomplish alone. For instance, if a therapist offers an explanation of your problems which you reject as ridiculous, then this might make it very difficult for you to continue one-to-one treatment with him. You might no longer trust his judgment, even if his interpretation is right. But in group therapy, if the other members of the group agree with the therapist's analysis of your problems, you cannot very well accuse them all of being biased or wrong. There is more evidence that the interpretation is right.

Group therapy also helps you to build up your confidence and break down the isolation which anxiety or depression might make you feel. It also gives you a chance to help others overcome their problems, something which can make you see your own in a new light.

PSYCHOANALYSIS

As I have said, most people tend to think of psychiatrists primarily as specialists in psychoanalysis, the technique devised by probably the most famous psychiatrist of all – Sigmund Freud. Freudian psychoanalysis can be very lengthy, lasting for two or three years before success is achieved, and is also very expensive. Even if you or your doctor doesn't feel it is the right approach for you, it is worth knowing about because Freud's theory of how the mind works gives us some insight into how anxiety or depression can sometimes result, and how they can be overcome.

What it is based on

Freud believed that most emotional problems and mental illnesses came from a part of the mind which he called 'the unconscious'. By this he meant the unconscious or subconscious mind from which we cannot recall memories at will, but which is the brain's store-house for formative childhood experiences and memories that can affect our daily lives if they have been unpleasant or unsettling.

He also felt that our conscious minds could only keep going – and on an even keel – by repressing the unconscious and its unpleasant memories. He believed that the conscious mind developed defences against the unconscious, and that in most people the unpleasant memories only surfaced in dreams which he felt were a sort of safety valve. They allow the mind to 'let off steam' in a harmless way from time to time, but even then the memories or unpleasant thoughts which crop up in our dreams are disguised to be less threatening. Freud believed that this was why most of our dreams are incomprehensible.

Difficulties arise when the mind's defences break down and can no longer hold the unconscious in check. This might be because the painful experiences of your childhood were too disturbing or too powerful and eventually break through, or because some change in your circumstances makes it harder for you to cope. Freud believed that the conscious mind's defences would often be able to distort what was coming from the unconscious enough to make any problem mystifying. The result would be anxiety about something odd, or a mysterious, apparently uncaused anxiety or depression. The problem would be disguised because if the conscious mind allowed itself to understand what was really wrong, the shock would be too much to bear. The work of people like Freud, Adler and Jung was so influential that phrases like 'inferiority complex' have passed into common usage. All the same they are often used incorrectly. What is meant by the term 'complex' is a collection and combination of ideas on a certain topic – like feeling inferior – which is suppressed into the unconscious mind.

Take the case of Donald, a man who started suffering from anxiety and depression late in life. He had three disadvantages about which people tend to feel inferior in our society. He was short, overweight, and he was illegitimate. During his childhood and early adult years he had suffered much criticism and adverse comment about these things. He had also grown up in a children's home, so had no money on which to launch himself into life.

Nevertheless, he worked very hard and developed a successful business of his own from nothing. He compensated for his other disadvantages too, and was always witty and entertaining company. However, he was mean with his cash and very unpleasant to his wife, making her beg for housekeeping money. He also tended to brag about his successes and his material possessions.

He certainly never complained about being inferior, concentrating on his strengths and on improving on a bad start in life. Nevertheless, he had felt inferior in the past, and these feelings of inferiority had made him feel anxious and depressed. So he repressed them into his unconscious mind. Someone like this is no

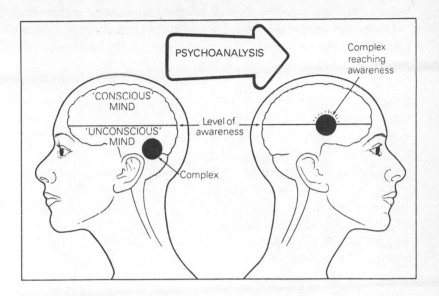

When a complex lies suppressed in the 'unconscious', it can cause mystifying feelings of anxiety and depression. Psychoanalysis aims to bring the complex into the conscious mind. This can be emotionally painful, but awareness often leads to recovery. (Note that this diagram is not meant to be an anatomical representation.)

longer consciously aware of feeling inferior – and Donald in particular was overcompensating, as his domineering behaviour shows.

In fact it would be fairly painful for someone like Donald if his feelings of inferiority were to come into his conscious mind – they would make him feel anxious and depressed again. So Donald was forced into the position of continually striving in his business and personal life to make sure that he was superior, not inferior. His behaviour was designed to prove that feeling inferior was the furthest thing from his mind.

But what happens if the repression of the complex begins to fail? In Donald's case, his business began to go badly. He found it hard to feel superior all the time, and so it was difficult for his mind to keep the complex repressed. It began to come to the surface, and started to make him feel tense and uncomfortable. Now that he could no longer avoid feeling inferior, he became extremely anxious and depressed – even more depressed than is usual in these circumstances.

Another way of putting this is to say that when a complex comes to the surface of the mind, it attacks your sense of well-being and self-esteem – and you feel vulnerable. The mind, as Freud described it, has a variety of defences against this sort of attack from within. Under certain circumstances, repression can again be used as a defence.

Other people use 'denial' as a defence. If Donald did this, he would continue to act in a superior and arrogant way, even though he no longer had anything to base his behaviour on – that is, no obvious successes. Others use what Freudian psychoanalysts call 'projection' – they blame others for their misfortunes, saying things like 'I'm not really inferior, my business failed because others conspired at my downfall out of jealousy.'

By using these defence mechanisms, the mind can banish the complex into the unconscious once more, and the sufferer will lose his anxiety or depression. This, though, can only be done at the expense of distorting reality. The problem is still there, in the sufferer's mind, and only needs another trigger to set it disturbing the conscious mind again.

How psychoanalysis works

I have already said that the sort of psychological help you can expect from your doctor – sympathy, reassurance, explanation, advice, suggestion, sympathy and encouragement – can be described as supportive psychotherapy. It aims to reduce the level of anxiety, and allows painful complexes or problems to subside once more into the unconscious.

Psychoanalysis, however, is often described as an 'insight-oriented' method of psychotherapy. It uses the processes of exploration, identifying and describing complexes, dealing with resistance to understanding, removal of defences, interpretation and the achievement of insight. We shall look at these aspects in detail in the following sections.

Exploration In psychoanalytic treatment, you will probably be asked to try to relax – perhaps by lying on a couch – and say whatever comes into your mind. You will be asked particularly not to hold things back because they are embarrassing or shameful – to be prepared, in other words, to tell the whole truth about what is going on in your mind, and not just the 'edited' version you normally divulge to others.

This process of letting ideas come out by themselves, one after the other, is called 'free association'. The aim is to reveal the strong feelings in the unconscious that can emerge in some form or other into the conscious mind, however well they are repressed.

In this sort of treatment, you will be the person doing most of the talking during the session. Talking takes up 90 per cent of the time you will spend with almost any type of therapist – and that means you talking. We have seen that just having someone to listen to you can be therapeutic in itself. Psychotherapists call this process 'ventilation', and it is close to what most people would describe as 'getting it off your chest'.

From time to time the analyst will ask you to tell him more about a certain topic – perhaps how you feel about your parents, for example. In this way, gradually and gently, the analyst explores the areas of your life which might be causing conflict. Sometimes there will be obvious matters of concern. You might say immediately that you are having problems with your job, and that you are sure this is where all your anxiety or depression stems from. On other occasions the source of worry might be more obscure, and the reason for your emotional upset will remain mysterious for the time being.

Often there are clues to the contents of the unconscious mind which the analyst can follow up. They may take the form of dreams, slips of the tongue or repeated patterns of behaviour. By discussing these in greater detail, the therapist carries out a process of exploration of your thoughts, designed to pin-point the sources of your trouble.

This sort of treatment might sound easy, but for some people the experience is quite difficult. You might even find that at the beginning it makes you feel even more anxious and tense – which is not what you had bargained for.

Removal of defences We have seen that defences of the mind against unpleasant feelings play a key role in the Freudian picture of anxiety and depression. Getting round these defences is an essential part of psychoanalysis.

Take the case of Donald, mentioned previously. He might go to see an analyst because he suffers from recurrent attacks of anxiety and depression, his defence mechanisms no longer being strong enough to cope with the surging of his complex towards his conscious mind. Though once the analyst begins to focus his attention on the things which cause Donald anxiety – his feelings of inferiority – his defences suddenly become very active and he develops a lot of resistance to what the analyst is doing. He does not actually want to think or talk about his real feelings – and that is his whole problem.

If the analyst gives up his attempt to explore these topics, respects Donald's resistance and even encourages him to repress the ideas once again, Donald might begin to feel comfortable; but he would not have made much progress. There is still the chance that he could suffer again.

Most analysts break through the resistance by pointing out the existence of the complex of unpleasant feelings of which someone like Donald may only have been partly aware. The analyst will say things like: 'You boast and brag because underneath you are really afraid of being inferior.' This process of revealing what was previously only in the unconscious mind is known as 'making an interpretation'. The analyst interprets Donald's behaviour and life history to show him what has been going on in his unconscious.

It is obvious that this process can be very uncomfortable. Donald will probably try to avoid accepting the interpretation. The skill of the analyst includes being right in his interpretation in the first place, of course, but also in enabling you to accept it and to obtain the benefit from seeing what is going on.

Insight The improved awareness of what is going on is called insight, and that is what gives its name to this sort of therapy. As Donald gains more insight into his mind, he may feel less compelled to brag. The analyst will be helping him to see that the things he thinks make him inferior are not so serious after all. Many people are short and overweight, and being illegitimate does not automatically make you a worse person.

With this sort of insight, Donald might be able to say: 'I might be inferior in some ways, but in other ways I am pretty good.' He will be ready to develop a more balanced outlook on life and concentrate in a better way on his strengths while expending less energy on repressing his complex. Facing what is going on in his unconscious mind will help to release him from its control and give him a better grasp of reality. This should help him to feel less anxious or depressed by his feeling of inferiority and build a better life for himself.

Of course the whole point of this treatment is to enable you to overcome problems like anxiety or depression by changing your behaviour or your attitudes or both. You will see that psychoanalysis has much in common with other forms of therapy, as well as obvious differences.

HYPNOSIS

In my experience this is the specialist treatment most people expect for their anxiety or depression. It has been much publicized in the media, and is attractive because it appears to provide a 'magic', effortless cure. In fact, it is very rarely used to relieve anxiety or depression – less than one person in a hundred receiving psychotherapy undergoes hypnosis. Although it is often extremely beneficial in pain relief, it is generally not so successful with emotional problems. It can, however, be useful in supportive psychotherapy for helping you to relax, or in insight-oriented psychotherapy to enable you to talk freely about your inner conflicts when you might find it too embarrassing or difficult to do so in a normal state of consciousness.

I mentioned briefly earlier on that we are all to a certain extent liable to the power of suggestion. If your doctor tells you firmly that he believes you will get better, then your chances of doing so are much higher, especially if you have confidence in his abilities.

Freud began his study of the mind and its problems with work in the field of hypnosis, and some psychoanalysts still use this technique to help them in their work with people who suffer from anxiety or depression, as do other therapists. There is nowhere that the power of suggestion works more effectively than in hypnosis.

Hypnosis is really an altered state of the mind, in which you are relaxed, more liable to suggestion, and in which things you might have repressed into your unconscious can be allowed to surface without causing you undue anxiety. During hypnosis you will probably be asked to lie on a couch to help you relax, and to fix your gaze on a point on the ceiling. The hypnotist will begin the process of suggestion by saying something like: 'As you relax, your eyes will start to feel tired.' He repeats a sentence like this monotonously and you will find it difficult to keep your gaze on that spot on the ceiling. Your eyes will start to feel tired, eventually giving a little flutter and closing.

There are no tricks, and nothing magical about hypnosis. Most people can be hypnotized, and some can even be made to regress to their childhoods. Some therapists claim even to have made people relive the experience of their own births, and the anxiety they felt on being expelled from the warmth and comfort of the womb into a cold, noisy and harsh outside world.

WHICH IS THE BEST THERAPY FOR YOU?

I have already said that few people can afford psychoanalysis. Few people would have the time or the determination to follow a complete course, either. This course involves an hour a day, five days a week for two or three years – and it often takes longer. It is very expensive, mostly because the analysts themselves have to undergo years of detailed training. So psychoanalysis is not usually available under health schemes, medical insurance, or national health services like the one in Britain.

I have gone into it in detail because it does play a part in other therapies, and less time-consuming forms of insight-oriented therapy have been devised to make it easier for people to obtain. One such method is to have the treatment sessions once a week instead of once a day, and aiming to have the course of treatment in eighteen months rather than three years. Clearly, less can be done in this way, especially if your problem is deep-rooted, but for many people this sort of course might be perfectly adequate.

So which therapy is the right one for you? Your first consideration will obviously be what is available to you, but close after this must come what demands a therapy will make on your time. If you are suffering from a mysterious depression for the first time in your life and it has only lasted a few weeks, then you would be right in thinking that it would be unwise to opt for a treatment which lasts several years.

In this case, your doctor's supportive psychotherapy might be all you need.

On the other hand, if you have had a long history of depression, and have tried tranquillizers, antidepressants and your doctor's psychological help, all with no apparent benefit, then you may really want to try and get to the bottom of your problems and sort them out once and for all. Some form of insight-oriented psychotherapy may well be your answer.

The other factor you should consider is whether you feel you can endure the discomfort of the process of exploration and removal of defences I described earlier in this chapter. We saw that this process can actually cause a temporary increase in your levels of anxiety and depression. If you decide that any further increase in your present degree of mental pain would be too much to bear, then insight-oriented therapies are not for you. You might feel, though, that a temporary increase in mental suffering is acceptable if it means a permanent solution to your problems. These decisions cannot be made lightly. If you do consider a lengthy course of treatment, it is essential to talk it over with a therapist beforehand.

Now that you know more about the different types of therapy available you can see that they all have their pros and cons. You might not be able to open up in group therapy, and feel the need for more personal, individual contact with your therapist. Behaviour therapy does not always work with people whose problems are deeply rooted in their minds; they simply might not be able to change their behaviour enough to make any difference. Supportive psychotherapies might not get to the root of your problems for the same reason – and there is then always the chance that the problem will resurface later on.

The picture is also slightly complicated by the fact that certain therapies can work in ways which they were not designed for. For example, in the course of talking in any therapy, certain things can happen. If you are having supportive psychotherapy, and you are becoming less anxious and more relaxed, with an increased feeling of security, then you might suddenly of your own accord develop real insight into underlying problems which you couldn't have borne to look at and examine earlier.

Similarly, if you are having insight-oriented psychotherapy, you might find that not only do you get an improved awareness of any underlying conflicts, but also that the process of talking to your analyst is a source of reassurance and encouragement for you – comforts which you would have thought more likely to come from supportive psychotherapy.

It is small wonder then that some therapists use what they call 'non-directive' counselling. In this, the therapist provides the opportunity for some simple 'ventilation' of your problems, with no predetermined goal. He or she will try to make you relaxed enough to get the benefits we have been talking about. In a way, this sort of free-flowing therapy allows you – almost automatically – to choose the approach that is best for you, whether it is insight or support.

Remember that most therapists will be happy to talk over their methods with you before you commit yourself to a lengthy course of treatment. With emotional problems like anxiety and depression, it is often difficult to tell what you need most until the treatment has actually been under way for a while. That is why some therapists may even recommend a few sessions of therapy on a trial basis so that you can both see whether his particular approach will be the best one for your situation.

8

ANXIETY AND
DEPRESSION IN WOMEN

WHY WOMEN ARE AT RISK

I have said that anxiety and depression can affect anyone at any time of life, but we know that women are generally more at risk. Indeed, some statistics show that around twice as many women as men are treated for these conditions, although it is likely that this is because women are probably more prepared than men to seek help. In Western society men tend to hide their feelings more, having been brought up to believe that 'big boys don't cry'. Most girls, on the other hand, are brought up to believe that it is right for them to show their emotions. The result is that women are more likely to talk about their feelings of anxiety or depression, while men tend to deny that they could be suffering in this way.

Several factors make women more at risk to anxiety and depression during their lives. I will be examining each of them in turn, but the obvious place to start is with the biological facts.

MENSTRUATION AND STRESS

One major difference between men and women is that women have periods each month and men don't. In basic terms, this means that there is a definite beginning and end to a woman's fertility. At puberty, there is the start of a girl's period, a time known as the menarche. If she is unprepared for this, it can be a deeply stressful event. Even when she knows that it is coming, and has had the whole process explained to her, it is still a major happening in her life – she has passed from childhood to adulthood in the space of a month.

Premenstrual tension (PMT)

Later on, she may have to face PMT. This is a very common experience, and involves both physical and psychological symptoms. If you suffer from PMT, you are likely to find that your mood changes just before your period. Around one woman in four feels anxious or depressed at this time, and you might also become irritable and perhaps even aggressive. Physically, your breasts, hands, ankles and feet may feel swollen up before your period, and at the same time your breasts may become tender. Many women also have stomach cramps actually during the time of menstruation. The effects of these symptoms – and women's attitudes to them – vary enormously from person to person. Some feel completely incapacitated with symptoms which others would ignore; sometimes a woman has deeper problems which cause her to focus on her feelings about menstruation and to experience the symptoms more acutely.

For some women, the symptoms – both physical and mental – become so distressing that as a result their relationships are damaged, their health suffers, and their ability to lead normal lives is seriously harmed. One major worry is that for most women menstruation is inevitable. It comes every month, and, if you are tense and anxious about the effects it might have on you, that tension will only serve to make it worse – and so on, in a vicious circle.

Several theories have been put forward as to why some women suffer from PMT. The most widely accepted is based on the fact that menstruation is controlled by the release of the two sex hormones, oestrogen and progesterone. These are released every month, and it is thought that the changes which they bring about in your body affect not only your sexual organs (they stimulate the ovaries to release an egg, and also the womb to develop a lining rich enough for a fertilized egg to embed itself in) but also other parts of the body, and your emotions too.

Why your attitude to menstruation is important   Girls are often brought up to think of menstruation as something dirty and unclean. Our society tends to look at all bodily secretions, like urine and faeces, in this way. There are taboos about our bodies which are reflected in our attitudes to certain acts we all have to perform – and in the fun we get from 'dirty' jokes. But menstruation is something which comes every month, it is unavoidable – so girls tend to grow up thinking that part of their natural functioning is dirty, and this causes tension.

Male attitudes to menstruation also play a part in creating tension in their partners. Few men know much about menstruation. 'It's something for women.' Some married couples never even discuss the subject, and rely on unspoken signals to work out when sex is 'permissible' and when it is not. In addition, some religions encourage people to believe that there is something wrong with sex during a period anyway. It is hardly surprising that all these social pressures can cause women to feel tense around the time of their periods.

Try to think of menstruation as a positive aspect of your life, as one essential part of a cycle – after all, without menstruation you could not have ovulation. This will go some way to removing the unnecessary aura of unpleasantness surrounding menstruation, and may help to reduce the tension, anxiety and depression you feel at this time of the month.

What else can be done?   There are treatments available which can often control and even cure PMT. Your doctor will probably recommend that you avoid any situations which might add to the stress on you in the few days before a period, and also that you take every opportunity to relax and enjoy yourself. Talking it over with a friend who has suffered in the same way will also be good therapy. Your doctor will also probably suggest that you try to keep your weight down to the level that is best for you which may in turn improve the hormone balance.

If you find that these methods do not help, your doctor may prescribe hormones to correct the balance in your body, perhaps recommending a spell on the contraceptive pill. Some types – known as the combined pill – contain oestrogen and progestogen, but there are other varieties, such as the progestogen-only-pill (POP), also sometimes called the mini-pill.

Drugs known as diuretics can also help to control the fluid in your body, and your doctor may prescribe tranquillizers to keep you calm and relaxed. The point to remember is that there is no need to suffer premenstrual tension in silence – your doctor can be asked for help.

ANXIETY AND DEPRESSION IN PREGNANCY

You might think that becoming pregnant is invariably a cause for celebration, and nothing else. For most women it is exactly that, but there are also aspects of being pregnant that can make you anxious and depressed.

The first of these is that however much you might want to have a baby, the actual fact of becoming pregnant may bring to the surface of your mind all sorts of doubts and uncertainties. You might begin to ask yourself questions like: 'Do I really want a baby?' 'How will I cope with the baby?' or 'Will I be a good mother?' Becoming a parent is a major change, and the confirmation of pregnancy puts a date to it – inevitably, you will have a baby and start a completely new and unknown part of your life. All this can provoke anxiety, and if the anxiety is not dealt with, you might become worried enough to be depressed.

In addition, a woman undergoes a number of physical changes which can be upsetting. Early on in pregnancy you can experience nausea and quite a lot of tiredness. This can lead to your feeling very run down – and not very happy about being pregnant. Added to this are the feelings of worry almost all mothers experience about the baby in the womb: 'Is the baby all right?' 'Is it normal?' or 'Will it be handicapped?' And most mothers – especially first-time ones – worry about the birth itself and how painful it will be, although this might be hard to admit to other people.

It is absolutely normal to have these feelings of anxiety, and you can do yourself a big favour by talking to other people who have been through it. Chat with friends or relatives, and you will find that most women will admit to being anxious during pregnancy.

What to do   Finding out as much as you can about pregnancy and childbirth could be a great help in dispelling your fears. Go to antenatal classes and learn the relaxation methods designed to help women cope with the pain of birth. These generally involve techniques of breathing, and could come in very useful in dealing with anxiety at any time of life. At antenatal class you will also meet other women in the same situation as you – and get support, sympathy and encouragement from them.

Pregnancy can also be a stressful time for fathers, and it is important for couples to communicate their feelings to each other during pregnancy. When both of them might be feeling anxious, unexpressed worries and negative thoughts can swiftly turn into resentments and brooding. Many couples find that they start arguing during a first pregnancy in particular, and this is because with all that worry and depression it is easy to turn on the nearest person – who might also appear to be the cause of the trouble in the first place.

When to seek help It is vital, however, to seek help from your doctor if you find that your anxiety or depression is becoming an overwhelming feature of your pregnancy. Your doctor will be able to help you to sort out whatever it is which is causing you anxiety, although to avoid any risk to the foetus he is highly unlikely to prescribe drugs for you in early pregnancy (see pages 58–9).

POSTNATAL DEPRESSION

The 'baby blues'

Most mothers experience postnatal (or postpartum) depression of one sort or another. Depression after the birth of a child can vary from a mild case of the 'baby blues' – which is very common – to a much rarer and more serious condition which I shall be covering later on in the chapter. It is estimated that over 50 per cent of mothers are depressed to some degree in the early days after birth, and this may be slightly more likely if it is your first baby or you have suffered regularly from premenstrual tension.

Why they happen Again, those powerful female hormones oestrogen and progesterone have been blamed for postnatal depression. Directly after birth there is a massive fall in the amount of hormones in a woman's body. She no longer needs them as their purpose was to provide the right environment for her baby in the womb. There is, however, virtually no evidence as yet to confirm that these hormone changes actually cause the depression.

There are probably other factors to be taken into account, too. The classic example of a mild case of baby blues is a feeling of weepiness, fatigue and apathy which comes over a woman on the second or third day after birth. Many women find then that they can be reduced to tears by even the most innocent comment. Part of this reaction comes from the sense of anticlimax which all of us feel after any long-awaited event – and pregnancy is after all a lengthy waiting period. Added to the changes in her hormone levels the new mother also has to cope with being tired and perhaps sore after all her exertions.

In recent years attention has been focused on the experience of birth itself as a factor in producing feelings of depression. For many mothers today, childbirth can be a highly technological and impersonal affair. Mothers are often made to feel as if they have a disease, rather than that they are women going through a perfectly natural process. For example, many mothers give birth to their babies in hospital delivery rooms which look more like operating theatres than anything else. They may be wired up to foetal monitors, their babies may be extracted by vacuum pumps or forceps, and many mothers are given episiotomies – that is, the skin near the vagina is cut to make more room for the baby to come out. Some campaigners for 'natural' childbirth have criticzed all this 'medicalization' of birth, and have also had strong words to say about giving mothers too many pain-killing drugs.

Another point of criticism has been the separation of mother and baby after birth. The campaigners say – and there is much evidence to back them up – that it is vital for mother and baby to be allowed time together immediately after birth so that 'bonding' can take place. This is the process whereby mother and child get to know each other and lay the foundations for their future relationship. It has been shown that the better bonding is, the easier it will be to get that relationship off to a good start. But often in hospitals the baby is taken away to be cleaned and weighed, and if the mother is heavily drugged she may not be able to communicate her wishes clearly.

The result is that many mothers feel that they had very little to do with the birth of their own children, that it was 'managed' and controlled by other people. Becoming a parent is difficult enough, as we shall see, without the added burden of a bad start. Childbirth can be an even more traumatic event if it is long drawn out or painful.

Getting over them   The good news is that times are changing. More and more obstetricians and maternity hospitals are working to make birth a much more satisfying experience for mother, child and father. Having your partner there while you give birth is good for all of you – it gives the mother someone she loves to support her, and gives the father a chance to do some of his own bonding, too. The 'baby blues' normally clear up of their own accord, and usually respond well to sympathy, reassurance and encouragement anyway. Most mothers feel much better about life within a few days, and simply knowing that what they are experiencing is a common reaction which will pass can be a great relief. If you know it might happen, then it will not seem so mystifying. It is also vital before birth to learn how to relax during your pregnancy, and to find out as much as you can about what childbirth is going to be like. Being prepared will help to make the experience less of a shock – and staying in control of what goes on during the birth itself, as well as actively trying to enjoy it, will make the experience richer and more rewarding. Talk things over with your doctor and try to let him know that you want your birth to be a good experience – he will probably be very sympathetic.

Depression in early parenthood

I said in Chapter 3 that the major changes in our lives are stressful events which can often cause anxiety or depression. Parenthood is no exception. As you move from the settled, comfortable status of being single or a childless couple to that of being a parent, you might become very anxious about how you will cope with your new responsibilities and unknown status; and once the baby has arrived you might feel low-spirited about the loss of some of your previous freedom.

Not being prepared   An additional problem is that in today's Western society very few parents have any real experience before the event of what having children is going to be like. In past centuries, when many families lived together in small villages or towns, and families were bigger, daughters would have had the chance to see how their younger brothers or sisters were born and brought up. They would have had the experience of helping mothers cope with the younger children.

When they became parents themselves, they would have been able to turn to their own mothers and grandmothers for help and advice, as well as to sisters, aunts and cousins. But the extended family of former generations no longer exists in our society. Most families have two or three children at most, and these are usually born at close intervals, so older sisters do not have the chance to see what bringing up children is like at close quarters. By the time they are old enough to learn from the experience they have forgotten it. Many families also live long distances away from relatives, so family help is no longer close at hand.

Furthermore, boys are not generally encouraged to gain any

experience of child-raising either. In most families, girls are given dolls, and boys are given other sorts of toys to play with – like footballs, guns or bicycles. The result is that many young husbands have got even less experience of babies and children than their wives, and however hard they might want to help, they simply do not know how to.

There are other, more direct, social pressures that can leave you badly prepared for parenthood. On the one hand, women are bombarded with advertisements and media features telling them that babies are beautiful and that parenthood is wonderful. They are also exposed to images which urge them to be gorgeous and seductive, too. There is much less emphasis in the media on how hard being a parent can be – on the sleepless nights, the feeling of total responsibility for this defenceless new being, the financial stress of having three mouths to feed on one person's salary.

The inevitable result for many women is that parenthood comes as something of a shock. Despite the fact that you buy the nappies or diapers which are supposed to keep your baby's bottom clean and dry, he still keeps you awake screaming half the night. Fathers too suffer from this sudden burst of reality, and may even resent suddenly getting less attention. Many a marriage goes through a very rocky phase in the early years of parenthood, with both partners tense, arguing and gloomy.

Isolation is another factor which can make life depressing for mothers, especially those who have just had their first baby. Most mothers still give up work and stay at home to look after the baby, and this can mean a dramatic change in lifestyle. It might seem that one moment you are at work, surrounded by friends and colleagues, and the next you are at home with no one but your baby to talk to. Add this to the factors I have already described, stir in some anxiety about whether you are a 'good' mother or not, and you have a good recipe for depression.

How to survive parenthood
There are several ways in which you can minimize or even avoid the anxieties and depression that can arise at this stage of your life.

1. Be prepared   If you have not had children yet, just reading this will help to counter those images of beautiful babies and happy parents you see all around you. Be prepared – parenthood is hard work and can be a strain. You will only get the best out of it – and it can be enormously rewarding – by knowing what you are letting yourself in for.

2. Try to get out   If you give up work to look after your baby, try to make some friends in your local area. Don't forget that there are probably hundreds of young mothers just like you who need a friend – you will meet them at your clinic, at antenatal classes before you have your baby, and at your doctor's. Do not be shy in coming forward – adult company is important.

There are also many different organizations which aim to bring mothers together and break down this isolation, such as Meet-A-Mum and the National Childbirth Trust in Britain. Find out about these and go along (see Chapter 11 for addresses). In many areas there are also nursery groups, mother and toddler groups and playgroups for your children – they are also good places to make friends.

Remember that you and your partner both need a night out from time to time – so find a babysitter and go. It is easy to put it off when you are tired and under pressure. But it is vital to enjoy life together, and doing so could play a large part in staving off depression.

3. Be honest about your feelings   Most parents feel negative about their children from time to time, and no wonder – they change your life forever. But don't be guilty about admitting to these feelings, even if they are very hostile. If you talk about it with other parents, you will find that most feel the way you do occasionally – suppressing your feelings may only make you depressed.

4. Seek help   If you ever feel that life is getting on top of you, and that you are really low, seek help. Just as with any form of depression, there is no need to suffer in silence – your doctor, community nurse or health visitor, or even just a friend might be able to help you.

Serious postnatal depression
The sort of depression and anxiety I have been describing is very common, but there is a more serious form of postnatal depression which has been estimated to affect 1 in 500 women after birth.

This is a serious depression – which has all the features of depressive illness I described in Chapter 2 – that comes on after childbirth. It most commonly happens after the birth of a first baby, but can occur after subsequent births, even if depression wasn't experienced previously. There is still much debate about its possible causes, and although hormone changes have been singled out, again there is no hard evidence to show that there is a connection.

The symptoms   are like those of severe depression in other circumstances (see Chapter 2). A woman might become very pessimistic and fear that she has a serious disease, or that her baby is handicapped in some way, continuing to believe this even when the doctor reassures her it is not so. She will also probably feel guilty and unworthy, and that she cannot possibly be a good mother. Some women even think that they will harm their baby in some way, perhaps breaking his neck when they hold him. Lack of energy and concentration, insomnia, a general feeling of sadness and gloom – sometimes even despair – are also common.

It has been known for some women to be so despairing that they feel life is no longer worth living. Fortunately, as a rule they are too lacking in initiative to attempt suicide, but a number have tried to kill their babies – to save them from 'this wicked world' – and themselves, and in some cases they have succeeded. That is why it is so important for them to get treatment as soon as possible.

Even if the woman does not attempt suicide, her feelings can still have a devastating effect on her life, health and family. I have said that depression impairs personal relationships, and nowhere is this to be seen more clearly than in postnatal depression. A husband might suddenly find that his formerly happy wife is now a completely different person, and she may find it very difficult to relate to her baby at all.

How it's treated   Even though we do not know what causes this form of depression, it can still be treated successfully. Many cases clear up satisfactorily with antidepressant drug treatments (see Chapter 6), but in the most serious, mothers are admitted to a hospital where they can be carefully watched during their treatment. In some areas there are special mother-and-baby units where parent and child can be kept together. It is important for the mother and child to have some contact with each other, if possible, for as we have seen, complete separation would only make the eventual reunion a more stressful event. Of course in cases where the mother is likely to harm her baby, doctors have to make very sensitive judgments as to how much contact there should be; but some, however little, is important – even if a nurse has to be present all the time.

Physical treatments for postnatal depression include the use of drugs and electroconvulsive therapy (ECT), which I shall be looking at in Chapter 10. ECT is particularly useful where a woman is so depressed that she feels suicidal, and prompt action is needed as a matter of urgency. Even if ECT is used as the main form of treatment, antidepressants are also likely to be prescribed (see pages 64–5).

One problem is that some women who suffer from postnatal depression do so while they are breastfeeding their children. There is a chance that small amounts of the antidepressant drug they take will get into the breast milk. If this would be harmful to the baby, then doctors would advise that the mother gives up breastfeeding while on the pills. As with all antidepressant drug treatments, it is important for the sufferer to keep taking the pills until the problem is overcome – this is to avoid a relapse, which could be very disheartening.

For some cases of postnatal depression drugs are not prescribed. Instead, psychotherapy is recommended, often of the supportive type which I described in the last chapter. In these cases the problem is often one of poor adjustment to family or circumstances. Psychotherapy will help the woman to talk through her problems and find her own solutions, whether it is a change in attitudes – looking at things in a different light – or adapting by living her life in a different way.

Even if you have suffered from a serious postnatal depression once, then you are still only slightly more at risk of suffering from it again after a subsequent birth. That is to say, the chances are still that you will not have a depression after the next delivery, and in any case you will be kept under careful observation for any emotional problems next time you are pregnant.

MISCARRIAGE, STILLBIRTH AND ABORTION

Sadly, not all pregnancies end successfully with the birth of a healthy child. Some women lose their babies earlier on in a miscarriage, which doctors call a spontaneous abortion. In recent years doctors have paid more attention to women's feelings after a miscarriage – and they are very often depressed.

The reason is simple. Even when a miscarriage happens very early on in pregnancy, a woman has still lost a child and will probably feel the need to grieve. In the past, women have often been told to 'forget about it', and try for another baby as soon as possible. Nowadays, though, we believe that women should be allowed to go through the process of mourning their babies. Suppression of their feelings may only lead to a more serious depression later on.

This is especially so in cases of stillbirth, where a woman may have gone through all the exertions of birth. Until recently, mothers were often not allowed to see or touch their dead babies, who were 'disposed of' by the hospital without the parents knowing how. Many doctors now believe that women should be offered the chance to see their babies so that they can have some focus for their grief, and that the babies should be buried or cremated with the full knowledge of the parents. In this way many questions which a mother might torment herself with in the following months will be answered, and she can mourn in the right way for her at the appropriate time.

Having an abortion by choice can also lead to depression, and this is something more people need to be aware of. Even a woman who has no trouble making such a decision may feel some sadness. Again, these feelings need to come to the surface to prevent a more serious depressive illness later on. Many women, though, have an agonizing time deciding whether or not to ask for an abortion. For them it is very important to obtain skilled guidance and counselling before coming to a definite decision. This advice should be sought as a matter of urgency, as this is a situation where the days and weeks available for discussion are strictly limited.

THE MENOPAUSE AND DEPRESSION

I said at the beginning of this chapter that there is a definite beginning to a woman's fertile life in the form of the first period, or menarche. There is also a definite end, and this is called the menopause.

Most women have their last period some time in their late forties or early fifties, although it can come later or earlier. For some women this end to fertility causes no difficulties at all. But for others –

and the figures may be as high as 75 per cent of all women – the menopause can be accompanied by unpleasant symptoms, both mental and physical.

What are the symptoms?

The common symptoms include sweating, hot flushes, dryness of the vagina and palpitations. You can also suffer from depression and anxiety with all their accompanying symptoms – like irritability, lack of energy and initiative, loss of concentration, insomnia and feelings of unworthiness and guilt. As with other forms of anxiety and depression, women may not experience all of them together to the same extent, but suffer more from insomnia and a feeling of sadness, for example, accompanied by one or two of the physical symptoms. Again, bodily changes have been blamed for some – if not all – of these symptoms. In the years preceding the menopause, your body does begin to change internally. The monthly rhythm of your cycle is disrupted as your ovaries work less efficiently, and this will affect the amount of hormones in your system as well as the duration and regularity of your periods.

Other factors

The menopause often comes at a time of life when a woman's children are growing up and about to leave home, or have already done so. If you have devoted your life to your family, you may feel that you now have nothing of value left in your life. Middle age can be a difficult time for a man, too – when he realizes that he can go no further in his career, for example, or that he is growing old. For married couples with children – and particularly for women – it can be a time of painful reassessment, a time to wonder what they can do with the rest of their lives. It is, perhaps, a case of grieving over the loss of a comfortable and known status again, something like moving from being single to being married, from being childles to being a parent. The menopause is symbolic of the end of a woman's role as a full-time parent with definite responsibilities and cares. Many women feel very anxious about their children leaving home, partly because they worry about them, but also partly because it is an end to one part of life; and many parents feel depressed after a child has married.

What can you do?

The self-help ways of overcoming anxiety and depression I discussed in Chapter 3 will also help you if you are having problems during your menopause. Sympathy and reassurance from a friend who has been through it all can be very helpful. Getting a break, giving yourself some pleasure in life, finding something to occupy yourself like a hobby or a new career can also be excellent ways of overcoming this sort of depression.

Above all, try to look on the positive side of the menopause. It is a time of life when you have more time and freedom to do what you want, rather than having your whole day taken up with routine family responsibilities.

What your doctor can do

If none of this helps, don't be afraid to go to your doctor – he will be able to help you. He will examine you to make sure there is nothing else – like a physical illness – which is causing your symptoms, just as he would anyone else with anxiety or depression. He may try to give you some supportive psychotherapy (see Chapter 7), and will certainly be able to help you with some of the symptoms, perhaps prescribing a lubricant to ease a dry vagina, or giving you some tranquillizers to help you sleep.

He can also give you hormone-replacement therapy (HRT), which will help to control troublesome or irregular periods, hot flushes and sweating by bringing your hormone balance back to its pre-meno-pause condition. Again, the hormones used are oestrogen and progestogen. You will probably have to take the it for several months, and your doctor will gradually cut down on the dose until you are ready to give them up entirely. He will not take you off them until he is satisfied that your menopausal changes are complete and your system has settled down. Of course, if your depression does not respond to this sort of treatment, then your doctor may well prescribe antidepressants (see Chapter 6), or even refer you to a psychiatrist (see Chapter 7).

9

OVERCOMING A PHOBIA

I mentioned phobias in connection with anxiety in Chapter 1, and said that they were a special form of fear, often the result of one anxiety-provoking situation which leaves a kind of 'emotional scar'. In this chapter I shall be looking at them in a little more detail, and also explaining how they can be overcome.

EXCESSIVE FEARS

There are many different types of phobia, but all of them have certain things in common. They are all irrational fears, or fears which are out of proportion to the circumstances.

We all have fears. Some of us are afraid of heights; others are frightened of spiders or elevators. Most of us accept these fears as normal and put up with the anxiety they cause, or take steps to avoid the things which frighten us. Some of us also have excessive fears; some people are very frightened of spiders, for example, but put up with the anxiety because it does not affect their ability to live normal lives. They may be paralysed with fear when they actually come into contact with a spider – and need the help of someone else to get rid of it – but for most of the time they are not anxious at all, mainly because the object of their fear is not around.

If you were to become so afraid of spiders that you felt you could not move out of one particular room in your house in case you met one, then you would have a phobia – in this case known as arachnophobia, an irrational fear of spiders. Being this frightened of spiders will make your life very difficult.

A phobia is, therefore, the name given to a disabling fear which stops you doing important things. Some phobias are worse than others, of course. If you are claustrophobic, for instance – which means being afraid of enclosed spaces – you might not want to use elevators. This could be a major handicap if you lived on the seventeenth floor of your apartment block and your office was on the twentieth floor of another building. Though if you lived and worked at ground level it might not be so disabling after all.

DIFFERENT TYPES OF PHOBIA

There are many different varieties of phobia. I have mentioned arachnophobia and claustrophobia, but some people suffer from a fear of heights, which is called acrophobia, others are afraid of certain types of animals, such as dogs or cats, and so on.

Agoraphobia

One form of phobia which is very common is agoraphobia. This is usually defined as a fear of open spaces, but it is a little more complicated than that. It is worth examining in detail as it throws some light on how any type of phobia may be caused. It mostly affects young women who spend much of their time at home with the children. A woman finds that she dislikes going down to her local supermarket (as I pointed out earlier, the word 'agoraphobia' means 'fear of the market place'). Soon she might find it difficult to go out of the house at all, and feels panicky whenever she does. The result is that it becomes easier to stay at home – all the time.

When agoraphobia reaches this stage, it is very disabling, and can often seem mysterious to the sufferer and her family. If you ask someone who is suffering from agoraphobia why she feels this way, she will probably be unable to tell you. The nearest she will get to it is to say that she is afraid of collapsing or fainting in public, or just making an exhibition of herself.

It is widely accepted that agoraphobia is related to the sort of problems women have to face, which I discussed in the last chapter. Housewives who find themselves under pressure and isolated at home may withdraw from the outside world, particularly if they are shy to start with. They may feel depressed about their situation and their circumstances, and depression can increase the feelings of isolation and unworthiness. This can make them frightened of meeting other people outside their homes, perhaps other mothers who appear to be coping better.

Names of some phobias

Animals	*zoophobia*	Fish	*ichthyophobia*
Birds	*ornithophobia*	Foreigners, strangers	*xenophobia*
Cats	*ailurophobia*	Germs	*mikrophobia*
Crowds	*ochlophobia*	Horses	*hippophobia*
Darkness	*nyctophobia*	Heights	*acrophobia*
Death	*thanatophobia*	Outdoors	*agoraphobia*
Dirt	*mysophobia*	People	*anthropophobia*
Disease	*pathophobia*	Sea	*thalassophobia*
Dogs	*cynophobia*	Snakes	*ophidiophobia*
Enclosed spaces	*claustrophobia*	Spiders	*arachnophobia*
Fire	*pyrophobia*	Thunder	*keraunophobia*

It is clear that a woman suffering like this is unable to lead anything like a normal life. She may be anxious and depressed most of the time, and her relationships with the rest of her family will be made very difficult – for they will have to do everything involving the outside world for her. She will also be unable to enjoy life, because she cannot go out, and may even find it very hard to venture out to her doctor for treatment. Professional treatment, though, is what everyone with a disabling phobia needs, and happily it is usually successful. So it is definitely worth making the effort to go and see your doctor; but if you really find it impossible to go outside the house, don't hesitate to ask him to make a home visit – he will understand.

HOW YOU CAN BE HELPED

There are several forms professional treatment can take. Your doctor may give you tranquillizers to help you deal with the anxiety the phobia causes, and if you suffer from agoraphobia he may use tranquillizers in combination with antidepressants to deal with your depression (see Chapters 5 and 6).

However, the most common form of treatment for phobias is a type of psychotherapy called behaviour therapy, which I mentioned in Chapter 7. Many psychologists believe that phobias are a type of learning which has gone wrong – a conditioned reflex which has no value, and which can spoil your life. The two methods that I am about to describe are techniques which have been developed by psychologists to help you unlearn those reflexes. Both are part of behaviour

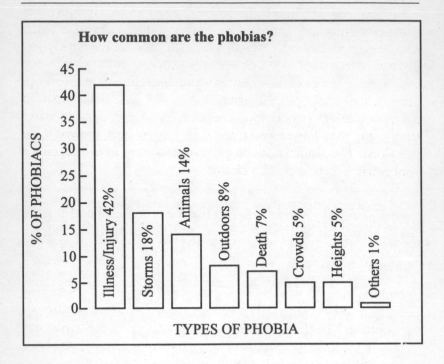

therapy and both are successful for around nine out of ten people who have them. The first is called 'desensitization', and the second 'flooding'.

The desensitization method   If you are suffering from a serious phobia, then this is the therapy you are most likely to be offered. It will be less traumatic than the flooding method, although desensitization will take longer to work. First of all you will be asked to draw up a list of situations which might be frightening, and then to put the list in order, with the most frightening at the top, and the least anxiety-provoking at the bottom.

The next step is to learn how to relax. This is usually done by helping you to achieve deep muscular relaxation with the sort of technique I described in Chapter 3. You will then be asked to imagine the least frightening situation on your list. As soon as you feel any anxiety, you stop and go through the process of relaxation again.

In time you will reach the stage where you can imagine that situation without any distress at all. At this point you can go on to the next item on the list and go through the same process. Eventually you become desensitized to the object of your fear – at least when you conjure up an image of that object in your mind. The next stage is to go through the whole process again, but in real life. Someone with agoraphobia, for example, might be taken by a helper on short walks from home, then longer walks, and then little by little allowed to do this alone. The example of one girl's success story in overcoming a phobia will help to make this clearer.

Yvonne was a thirteen-year-old schoolgirl who was very frightened of birds and feathers – a rare type of phobia. It started at the age of eight, when a pigeon flew up in her face while she was walking through a park on her way to school. After this incident she stopped going through the park and took a longer route to school through a built-up area. If she saw a bird approach, she would try to hide under a parked car or dash across the road, oblivious to traffic.

Although her fear of birds was interfering with her life, she was able to get by until a traumatic incident occurred three years later. Her fellow pupils were rehearsing for a Christmas play, which involved using a feather duster as a prop. Yvonne screamed and fled immediately when this object appeared. After this the other children, in teasing mood, would chase her with the duster and hide feathers in her desk. She stopped going to school and eventually was referred to a clinical psychologist. It was decided to treat her with desensitization.

A list was drawn up of situations that she found difficult, ranging from gazing at a sparrow's feather 10 ft (3 m) away, to feeding the pigeons at Trafalgar Square in London. She was given some training in relaxation and exposed to each of the situations in real life, accompanied by the therapist. This involved showing her feathers of different shapes, colour and size which were brought closer and closer until she could touch them without any distress. She was then shown slides and films of birds and encouraged to imagine herself approaching them. A visit to the aviary at London Zoo followed soon afterwards.

The planned visit to Trafalgar Square took place on the twelfth session, and she experienced only slight anxiety while feeding the pigeons. The therapy was ended at this stage and she was able to return to school. She could cope quite easily with attempts made by her fellow pupils to frighten her. Three years later, she was still free from the phobia and was enjoying life to the full.

With the desensitization method, anything from ten to thirty sessions of treatment might be needed to overcome the phobia.

The flooding method

This type of behaviour therapy is more or less the direct opposite of desensitization. In this, you will be allowed to become anxious and then work through the distress. You are exposed to the feared object or situation, and the contact is kept up for hours until your anxiety wears away.

This way you will learn that nothing horrible actually happens, and the object will lose its terror for you. As with desensitization, flooding can be carried out in your imagination first, and then in reality. Although it will be stressful, it can often be a better choice of therapy for those people who need urgent help with their phobias, as the case of Jean shows.

Jean was a thirty-year-old social worker who had an acute fear of heights – acrophobia. She felt very uneasy when she went above the third floor of an apartment block. She could remember quite clearly how the problem began. At the age of six she had been chased by a dog on an upper floor of a large department store. She had pressed herself against a plate glass window in a state of panic and looked down. From then on she had her acrophobia.

Her fear of heights interfered with her life because it meant she was not able to see a large number of the clients allocated to her. In fact, when she was referred for therapy, she was in grave danger of losing her job. Because there was a degree of urgency here, it was necessary to use the flooding method rather than desensitization. Flooding can be an unpleasant form of treatment, but it is very effective.

In Jean's case, the therapist took her up in the elevator to the fifteenth floor of an apartment block, and encouraged her to stand close to the chest-high wall and look down. She immediately became very distressed and the therapist had to coax and cajole her into staying. It took two hours before all traces of anxiety disappeared. For another half an hour, while in a weary state, she was encouraged to remain looking down from the wall. Her therapist continually pointed out, during this stage, that although she was in the worst possible anxiety-provoking situation for her, she was not panicking.

The next morning, the therapist took Jean up again and, apart from some twinges of anxiety during the first twenty minutes, she felt quite relaxed. She was kept up there for a further hour. It was decided that she needed no more treatment after this. The therapist saw Jean several times over the next five years to see how she was doing, and at no time did she find that her phobia had returned.

As you can see, phobias can be treated successfully, and it's worth repeating that nearly everyone who is treated with either of these two types of psychotherapy will be rid of their phobia for good. What happens, though, when someone is so tense or depressed that life becomes unbearable, and he or she feels that something drastic has to be done? In the next chapter we shall be looking at just how serious a problem this can be and what can be done about it.

10
WHEN LIFE CAN SEEM UNBEARABLE

For those of you who have never been made to feel desperate by depression, it might be difficult to put yourself into the mind of someone who is so depressed that life seems unbearable. We have all felt anxious or sad at times, but for most of us this is only a temporary problem.

If it comes for a long time and nothing seems to help, you can feel very depressed indeed. Nothing is going right, you feel very pessimistic about the future – and your pessimism seems totally justified. You cannot get out of your black mood, whatever you do. Eventually, the idea that you never will feel happier might occur to you. You start to think that things will never sort themselves out. You might begin to look back over your life through depression-tinted spectacles and wonder if any of it was worth while. Finally, you might begin to think of ending it all. You have reached the edge of despair.

Although it is a very painful state of mind to be in, many people get to this stage of hopelessness without doing anything drastic or irreversible. One of the protective mechanisms which stops them doing so lies in the fact that when you are that depressed you are also likely to be lacking energy and initiative. So although you might think of harming yourself – or committing suicide – you may well not have the drive to do so. I shall be examining the problem of suicide in detail in this chapter, but first let's look at one way in which you can be helped before you get to this stage.

ELECTROCONVULSIVE THERAPY (ECT)

Who might benefit from ECT?
ECT is a physical method of treatment for depression which has a very high rate of success. It might be offered to you before you get to the stage of total despair and thoughts of suicide, but because it is so

effective it is often used to treat people who feel they might want to kill themselves – in these cases, it is a treatment which actually saves lives.

It might also be suggested to you if you have been having drug treatment or psychotherapy which does not seem to be working. People who cannot cope with the side-effects of drugs might also be better suited to ECT, as well as those who might not feel suicidal but who have reached the stage of 'nervous breakdown'. This is not a phrase doctors tend to use, unless it is to persuade someone that they need treatment when they might be reluctant to accept it. But you can get to the stage with depression where normal life becomes totally impossible and you need drastic help – which is a good definition of the way the phrase 'nervous breakdown' is used by most people. Endogenous depressions – those that occur for no obvious reason – often do better with ECT, too.

What exactly is ECT?
ECT is a therapy which involves passing a small electric current through the brain. This causes you to have a convulsion, much the same as an epileptic fit. ECT is done in hospital, and you will be given a general anaesthetic – so that you will not actually feel anything while it's being performed. A special substance will also be injected to relax your muscles, so that you cannot hurt yourself during the fit. The shock is actually administered through two electrodes which are placed on the side of your head. The whole procedure takes only a few minutes, and you will be awake within a quarter of an hour or so.

Are there any side-effects?
You can feel sleepy after a session of ECT, and some people have aches in the muscles and headaches as well. You could also be a little vague and have trouble remembering things. Most of these effects wear off fairly soon – usually in a day or two.

It is important to tell the doctor who is giving you the treatment about any drugs which you might be taking – this is because the drug which the anaesthetist uses to get you off to sleep could interact harmfully with others in your system, such as a MAOI-type antidepressant, for example (see Chapter 6).

How soon does ECT start producing results?
You will probably be offered two or three treatments per week to start

with, and you should be feeling noticeably better by the time you have had four or five. How many treatments you will need before you are completely better depends on you, and the doctor who is treating you will keep a close eye on your progress so that he can make the best decision; but it is rare to need more than twelve.

How effective is ECT?

We still do not know exactly why ECT works, but it is very effective, relieving depression in around nine people out of ten who have the treatment. It is sometimes used in combination with other treatments like drugs and psychotherapy, but even on its own it has cleared up depression in very many people. Some people are very frightened at the prospect of having an electric current passed through their brains, but it has been shown to be very safe. In cases where life is unbearable, it can literally be a life-saver. All the same, its use has been banned or severely restricted in some European countries and States of the USA. In view of the good it can do and its acceptable safety record, I believe that the voices raised against it are mistaken. Clearly everyone has to make up their own mind.

SUICIDE

It is unfortunately true that there are still a lot of people who are suffering from a degree of depression that seems unbearable. Perhaps they don't seek help, and therefore never get the chance to help themselves or use antidepressants. Even so, to think of killing yourself is a very drastic step – and most people need another factor to push them over the edge, without which they will remain resigned to their feelings and continue to suffer in silence.

Most commonly, this other factor is desperation. When you get to the stage of being desperate, you will probably feel that you cannot bear to suffer a minute longer. You might experience a sense that something decisive has to be done – immediately. Often this feeling of desperation can be triggered off by an event that crops up unexpectedly. You might suffer a sudden disappointment, someone might make you feel rejected or a relative might say something hurtful and wounding. This could be the straw that breaks the camel's back.

You might not attempt suicide immediately, though. Some people in their desperation go and get drunk, or do something destructive – like breaking a valuable possession, for example, or lashing out at someone they love. But an attempt at suicide is the form of action which some people take when they have reached this stage.

Not just a way of getting attention

There is a popular belief that people who talk about suicide never do it. The idea behind the belief is that talking about it is just a way to draw attention to yourself, to worry other people, or to try and get your own way. There is certainly some truth in the idea that when someone feels hopeless and desperate they might want to draw the attention of others to their plight, especially if they feel that nobody understands. They might also feel angry towards other people, and want to do something dramatic to make them appreciate what they are going through. Revealing their suicidal thoughts might seem like the only way of prodding others into some form of response.

However, it is certainly not true that people who talk about it never carry out the final act. In fact, the opposite is true; someone who talks about suicide is much more likely to kill himself than someone who has never mentioned it. Such talk should be regarded as a danger signal, that the person needs help and expert advice. It is difficult to put an exact figure on it, but my own estimate is that someone who talks about – or even admits to suicidal feelings – is probably ten or even a hundred times more likely to kill himself than someone who does not.

To put this in perspective, the suicide rate in most countries works out to an average of about 1 death in 10,000 of the population per year. That means that if a vulnerable person has a hundred times greater chance of committing suicide than the average person, his chance is one in a hundred – which is pretty high.

Another popular belief is that people who try to kill themselves and fail 'did not really mean it', and that they are less likely to commit suicide. Someone who attempts suicide by taking an overdose and whose life is saved is often said to be trying to gain attention. Sometimes such attempts at suicide are written off as a 'cry for help'.

Again, exact figures are difficult, but one particular piece of research is very illuminating. Two American scientists in Philadelphia – J. Tuckman and W. F. Youngman – carefully followed up individual people who had been admitted to hospital after an attempt at suicide.

They wanted to find out which of them actually killed themselves in a subsequent attempt. They discovered that in the group of people they studied, the death rate from suicide was 150 times that of the general population. I think this shows clearly that people who attempt suicide are not just being dramatic. Far from their being less likely to kill themselves, they are much more likely to.

What are the risk factors?

Who else is at risk from suicide other than those who have talked about it or have actually attempted it? Much research has been done into this subject, and certain broad main categories can be outlined.

Your sex   More men commit suicide than women, but in recent years the relative numbers of women suicides has increased. Women are more likely than men to take an overdose of drugs.

Age   People who commit suicide are more likely to be elderly. This varies slightly from country to country, but in general, those over the age of sixty are more at risk.

Background   Suicides are more likely to have had a history of mental illness in the past. They are also more likely to have been dependent on drugs or alcohol. They are most often people who live in the centre of cities and who are alone, unmarried, widowed or divorced. Married people who commit suicide are often childless, and are the children of divorced or separated parents themselves. They may have been accustomed to a high standard of living, but are currently in reduced circumstances. Suicides are also more likely to be suffering from a physical disease.

Occupation   People particularly affected are doctors, dentists, lawyers and students. Often there has been a break in the pattern of their lives. This may take the form of retirement, loss of a job for other reasons, or bereavement. These are the sort of stress-laden events in life which I discussed earlier on – and they are also more common in the elderly.

Protective factors   Suicide is actually less common among those who have large families – especially a large number of children – and who are religious.

This list is useful in some ways, but not in others. If I met a retired, single lawyer living alone in the centre of a city who was suffering from a physical illness, I would not automatically assume that he was at great risk of committing suicide. On the other hand, if he had talked about suicide, or recently attempted it, then I would definitely consider him to be at risk. As with anxiety and depression, suicide is something which can happen at any time of life to anyone – given the wrong circumstances.

Who is most likely to carry it through?

Women are more likely to try to kill themselves and fail than men, and usually they are young – mostly in their late teens or early twenties. They often come from poor homes and work in relatively unskilled jobs. People who actually kill themselves are more likely to have been suffering from a serious level of depression for some time, while many of those who try and fail have had only a brief emotional upset.

Despite these differences, I believe it is a mistake to think that people who attempt suicide and those who actually kill themselves are completely different types. There is a lot of overlap between the two groups, and in terms of risk to life in suicide attempts you can see all ranges of overdose, for example, from very minor ones, to major ones where doctors have to make enormous efforts to save life. In the case of these near-fatal attempts, it is clearly a matter of chance or fate that the outcome was one of attempted suicide rather than death.

An epidemic of suicide

More and more people have attempted suicide in recent years, most commonly by an overdose of drugs. In some places, self-poisoning with a drug is the commonest cause of admission to hospital.

When I qualified as a doctor 40 years ago, the rates were about 3 attempted suicides per every 10,000 people in the population. Now the annual rate is more like 30. To put it another way, for every person who actually commits suicide, 30 people try, and most of these attempted suicides are women.

It is difficult to know exactly why there has been such a big increase in the rate of attempted suicide over the last few decades. It is unlikely that the amount of depression which people suffer from has increased by ten times. It could have something to do with the fact that far more drugs are prescribed these days – and so an easier form of attempted suicide is more readily available.

But I suspect that it is more related to the ways people are now less prepared to put up with depression than previously. Many people have heard that it is possible to overcome the problems, and feel frustrated if they do not get the right sort of help or treatment. This frustration might be the triggering factor that provides impetus to make the suicide attempt. Again, this puts the onus on all of us – family and friends as well as doctors and specialists – to make sure that we get help for anyone who is feeling this way.

Why those who want to commit suicide must be dissuaded

Most people with suicidal feelings can be helped so that they avoid killing themselves. However, there are those who believe that anyone who wants to kill himself should be allowed to do so – perhaps that they should even be helped in their attempt. I am very much opposed to this idea. In the course of my career I have been in contact with hundreds of people who have been depressed to the point of feeling suicidal. Almost always this feeling does not last. With support, they begin to feel better after a while and if they had been encouraged to end their lives at the point when everything felt unbearable, no doubt many would have done so – and this would have been an extravagant and tragic waste of life. I cannot emphasize too strongly that no matter how sincerely people believe at the point of crisis that the right thing to do is to end their lives, in the course of time they will lose their suicidal feelings and begin to enjoy life again.

You might say that there are exceptions, like people who have serious illnesses and only a short time to live. But I know that some people with diseases such as cancer, who are seriously depressed, feel much better if they get help for their feelings of sadness. They can come to terms with the prospect of death and find a certain amount of reward and pleasure in the life that remains to them.

Do seek help

Obviously, if you feel at all suicidal – whether or not you think you might be suffering from depression – then it is time to seek help urgently. It does not matter if the feeling is only temporary, it is still a sign that your mood has reached a dangerously low level. Talk it over with someone who you know will be sympathetic and enlist their support – and go to your doctor as soon as possible, or anyone else who might be able to help (see Chapter 11 for useful addresses).

Very often, people who have reached this stage have gone beyond the point where they seek help of their own accord. It is therefore vital that those around them should be able to recognize the symptoms and step in to avert a possible tragedy.

How to recognize a potential suicide

Even if you suspect that someone you are close to is contemplating ending it all, you still might hesitate to ask him or her directly. Often someone who is in such a frame of mind will tell you anyway, without waiting to be asked. But if not, do not hold back – if you are worried, ask about it; for the person who feels that way, just having someone to talk to about these terrifying feelings might be an enormous relief.

The main way of telling that someone is feeling suicidal is if they are obviously despairing and desperate. The two are not the same – the former means feeling hopeless, and the latter, wanting to do something drastic. If a person experiences both of these things at the same time, he or she is at great risk.

Some people are reluctant to admit that they are feeling suicidal. If their religious beliefs tell them that suicide is a sin – as is the case with Roman Catholics – they may even try to avoid admitting the feeling to themselves. Some in fact deny it right up to the time that they try to end their lives. Again, it is important to break through this reluctance – and also to get them in touch with support and expert help as a matter of urgency.

Others, even though they are loath to say they are feeling suicidal, will admit, though, that they do not positively want to go on living. They go to bed at night very depressed, and at that time they sometimes feel that they would not care if they never woke up. They might feel that taking their own life is repugnant and wrong, but that does not mean they want to stay alive; quite the contrary. These people need to be taken seriously, too – and given the treatment they so urgently require.

Helping someone who is plagued by suicidal thoughts

There are some simple things you can do which almost always help people who feel suicidal – and can even prove life-saving. You might be tempted to try some reassurance, but this doesn't always work. If you say: 'I have read that feeling suicidal is something which does not last,' your friend probably will not believe you, and feel that you do not really understand.

Talk things over   This is something which will be much more effective. Instead of suggesting to your friend that there is hope, you could encourage him to tell you how hopeless he feels. Instead of telling him to be patient, you can encourage him to tell you how impatient and desperate he feels.

In this way you will allow him to get things off his chest, and give him the satisfaction of really conveying to someone exactly what he is going through – somebody who listens and does not turn away or change the subject. This has two benefits. To start with, it is a relief to pour out your troubles when you are feeling low, as we have seen many times throughout the book. Second, if your friend feels that he has got his message across – that someone else does understand that he is feeling like ending it all – then he does not have to go ahead and prove it. Therefore he is less likely to make the attempt.

It is one of the basic principles of all counselling methods that if people can talk out their problems, this helps them to avoid acting them out. Of course, it is vitally important in this case – because acting out the problem could be lethal.

Arrange to meet your friend again   The time might come in a situation like this when you feel that you have to say something positive, offer some sort of solution; but we have seen that people who are very depressed often take advice or sympathy – as they do reassurance – in the wrong way. Or it might be that your friend's problems look enormous and insoluble.

In fact you don't have to suggest anything. You certainly don't have to offer wise or dramatic solutions. Instead you could offer to meet your friend once again – perhaps regularly – to talk things over. In effect, you will be throwing him a lifeline by letting him know that you will be available to help him. How soon you meet is a matter of judgment. If you think the situation is serious it could be later that same day; if less so, the next day or even the next week. You could give him your telephone number, or a way of contacting you when you are not at home. All this shows you care; and it also shows that you believe your friend will be around to come to your next meeting. After meeting again a few times, you might find that his suicidal thoughts disappear. Then you can be fairly certain that you have been instrumental in avoiding a crisis.

Encourage your friend to seek help If your friend is not already being treated by a doctor or therapist, try to persuade him to go along to someone who can help him. Again, he might be very pessimistic about this and reluctant to be persuaded, but it is vital he goes. It might do the trick if you offer to go along with him.

Make emergency arrangements just in case your friend tries to harm himself while you are absent. Something might crop up before you see him again which will make him really desperate – and it could be something trivial.

Giving him your telephone number is one thing you can do, but you should also make sure he has the numbers of his doctor, local hospital or social worker's department to hand too. Give him the numbers of other friends or relatives who might be able to help him, as well as any voluntary organizations you might know of in your area (see Chapter 11). Having all these numbers might save his life; if one number is busy or there is no answer when he is in desperate need of help, he can always try the next one. Warn people that he might telephone – especially family and his doctor. You could also phone from time to time, just to let him know you are still there to help.

How to cope with a crisis

You might be faced with a terrible dilemma if your friend lives on the tenth floor of his apartment block or has a cupboard full of pills. Supposing you are just about to leave him alone while you go and call the doctor or fetch extra help. What do you do?

It is best to ask your friend as tactfully as possible how he feels about being left in such potentially dangerous circumstances. He may not understand at first, but when he does, his answer might give you a clue as to the extent of his feelings. It might take one of three forms.

1. He might say: 'It's all right to leave me. I see what you mean, but I wouldn't do anything silly while you are going for help.' If this

is said in a normal tone of voice, this is an answer that you can probably trust. The right thing to do is to go for help – and accept your friend's word.

2. He might say: 'I wouldn't like you to go. I'm worried about what I might do to myself if you were gone too long.' Under these circumstances it would be wrong to go out and leave your friend alone. You will have to find some other way of dealing with the situation. You might have to persuade him to come with you.

3. Sometimes the reply is uncertain. 'Well, I'm not sure. I suppose I might be all right.' In this case, you should take no risks. Treat your friend as if he has said that he is not happy to be left alone.

Can people who feel this way be treated?

Treatment for people who feel suicidal is much the same as for people who are seriously depressed but who do not feel like ending their lives. ECT, which I described at the beginning of this chapter, and antidepressant drugs (see Chapter 6) are often used to good effect.

The danger is that treatment can actually restore enough initiative to someone who is feeling suicidal to make their next attempt successful. That is why people who have attempted suicide and who are receiving treatment are often kept under close observation: it is a particularly distressing tragedy to watch someone improving and then to see them end their lives. It is also something relatives and friends of the suicidal should keep in mind.

All the other methods I have described – like psychotherapy and other specialist help – can also be successful with people like this, depending on the causes of their depressions. The outlook is good for them: many thousands of people who have been brought back from the brink of suicide go on to lead full and normal lives.

11
WHERE YOU CAN GET HELP

In the course of the book I have already looked in detail at many of the most likely sources of help for your anxiety or depression: you yourself; your loved ones, family and friends; your family doctor, psychiatrists, psychologists and other qualified specialists.

In this concluding chapter I want first to draw your attention to the sort of aid other organizations and agencies can provide, and then to list some addresses that you might find useful.

SPECIAL AGENCIES AND ORGANIZATIONS

Social workers
In most countries there are social workers whose job it is to help people cope with a vast range of everyday problems. They can usually offer aid and advice in many areas such as money, poor housing, unemployment, family strife and so on. Many social workers are also trained in counselling and psychotherapy. In fact many people could be helped equally by a doctor or a social worker. Social workers are skilled at dealing with practical problems and offering a broad style of help. Although doctors can do this too, they are more expert at using physical treatments like drugs. Social workers can also refer you to more specialist help when it is needed – for legal or marital advice, or help with your children's education. You can approach them yourself, or ask your doctor to refer you to them.

Other health workers
Many countries also have skilled health workers other than doctors or hospital nurses: community-based nurses and health visitors, for example, who work in one particular district and who can also offer help and advice on a wide variety of health-related problems.

Community-based midwives and maternity nurses are often the first line of defence for women who suffer from postnatal depression (see Chapter 8).

Churches
Churches and religious institutions of all kinds have a long history of giving relief to people in distress. Many people who suffer from anxiety or depression may obtain a lot of help from their priests or ministers, church visitors or even just sympathetic members of the congregation.

Voluntary organizations
Churches have played a key part in the foundation and running of many of the voluntary organizations that exist to give support to people in difficulty. The Samaritans is one such organization and there are many, many more.

Groups like the Samaritans are best known for being available at the end of the telephone to help people who are feeling suicidal. They also give a great deal of assistance to people who are in trouble of any kind, but who may not be thinking of killing themselves. I have already discussed suicide in Chapter 10; suffice it to say here that groups like the Samaritans have saved many lives and relieved an enormous amount of distress.

Indeed, there are voluntary organizations, often manned by sufferers themselves, aiming to help people cope with just about every problem or condition. There are groups to help lonely and depressed mothers; women who have had stillbirths or miscarriages; people with skin diseases, heart disorders or diabetes. There are organizations to help alcoholics and their families – and, of course, to help those who suffer from anxiety and depression.

These types of agency can often offer specific advice on particular problems, as well as practical help. They can also help you to meet other people who have suffered – and survived – what you are going through. Your doctor, social services department or local council may be able to refer you to the particular group which would suit you, and they are well worth finding. Many of them will also be listed in your phone book, and organizations like the Samaritans also keep their own lists of helping agencies. I have included the addresses of some of the major ones at the end of this chapter.

Marriage guidance counsellors

If your anxiety or depression is related to a marital or sexual problem, you might try going to a marriage guidance counsellor. They are specialists who are trained to help you with difficulties in your relationship, and, as we have seen, these are the commonest causes of anxiety and depression. You do not necessarily have to be married to see a counsellor; so long as you have a stable relationship, they will probably be prepared to help you. A marriage guidance counsellor can recommend that you see a sex therapist, who is trained to deal with specific sexual problems – such as impotence, premature ejaculation and frigidity – which might cause distress between partners. These are often the result of anxiety – and may lead to further anxiety and depression.

Other helpers

Your local policeman may often be able to help you out. Perhaps one of your neighbours is making your life a misery with all-night parties and general hostility. A word from the police might make life a lot easier.

People also often go to their local pharmacist for his or her opinion on illnesses and ailments such as bad nerves or irritability. He or she may be able to give you some simple counselling, and advise you on any drugs which your doctor might prescribe for your illness (see Chapters 5 and 6).

USEFUL ADDRESSES

GREAT BRITAIN

Age Concern
Astral House
1268 London Road
London SW16 4ER
Tel: 0181 679 8000

Al-Anon Family Groups (for relatives of problem drinkers)
61 Great Dover Street
London SE1 4YF
Tel: 0171 403 0888

Aleph One Ltd (biofeedback)
The Old Courthouse
High Street
Bottisham
Cambridge CB5 9BA
Tel: 01223 811679

Association for Post-Natal Illness
25 Jerdan Place
London SW6 1BE
Tel: 0171 386 0868

British Association for Counselling
1 Regent Place
Rugby
Warwickshire CV21 2PJ
Tel: 01788 578328

British Association of Psychotherapists
37 Mapesbury Road
London NW2 4HJ
Tel: 0181 452 9823

Centre for Autogenic Training
15 Fitzroy Square
London W1P 5HQ
Tel: 0171 935 1811

Compassionate Friends
53 North Street
Bristol BS3 1EN
Tel: 01179 539639

Cruse Bereavement Care
Cruse House
126 Sheen Road
Richmond
Surrey TW9 1UR
Tel: 0181 332 7227

Depression Alliance
PO Box 1022
London SE1 7QB
Tel: 0171 721 7672

Depressives Anonymous
36 Chestnut Avenue
Beverley
North Humberside HU17 9QU
Tel: 01482 860619

Gingerbread (one-parent
families)
49 Wellington Street
London WC2E 7BN
Tel: 0171 240 0953

Manic-Depression Fellowship
8–10 High Street
Kingston-upon-Thames
Surrey KT1 1EY
Tel: 0181 974 6550

Meet-a-Mum Association
14 Willis Road
Croydon CR0 2XX
Tel: 0181 665 0357

**MIND (National Association
for Mental Health)**
Granta House
15–19 Broadway
Stratford
London E15 4BQ
Tel: 0181 519 2122

National Childbirth Trust
Alexandra House
Oldham Terrace
London W3 6NH
Tel: 0181 992 8637

The Phobics Society
4 Cheltenham Road
Chorlton cum Hardy
Manchester M21 9QN
Tel: 0161 881 1937

Relaxation for Living
12 New Street
Chipping Norton
Oxfordshire OX7 5LJ
Tel: 01608 646100

**The Royal College of
Psychiatrists**
17 Belgrave Square
London SW1X 8PG
Tel: 0171 235 2351

The Samaritans
10 The Grove
Slough
SL1 1QP
Tel: 01753 532713

**Seasonal Affective
Disorder Association**
PO Box 989
London SW7 2PZ

**Women's Therapy
Centre**
6 Manor Gardens
London N7 6LA
Tel: 0171 263 6200

INDEX

Other emotional well-being titles available from

VERMILION

ALL IN THE MIND?
Think yourself better
Brian Roet

Have you a problem that won't go away? This book offers a key to solving long-term problems, physical, social and emotional. Drawing on his practical experience, Dr Brian Roet shows how the mind plays a major role in causing and maintaining illnesses, and how many physical and psychological symptoms are messages from the unconscious.

By unravelling our thought processes and using practical self-help techniques, Dr Roet shows everyone how they can start on the road to self-knowledge and recovery.

PERSONAL THERAPY
How to change your life for the better
Brian Roet

In this book Dr Roet shows us how therapeutic techniques can be used to release deep-seated emotions, acknowledge our strengths and weaknesses and establish emotional equilibrium. His reassuring and practical advice guides us towards new ways to enjoy a more fulfilling life.

Case studies are used to reassure and advise readers of the benefits of personal therapy and how it can play an active role in helping the mind resolve anxieties and even disease.

BE ASSERTIVE
The positive way to communicate effectively
Beverley Hare

This book will introduce the reader to the techniques of assertiveness training, which can be invaluable in all areas of life.

Beverley Hare dispels the myth that assertive behaviour is aggressive, and draws on her own experience to explain how becoming more assertive can help us all to improve the quality of relationships, both in the business environment and in our personal lives.

SEX: HOW TO MAKE IT BETTER FOR BOTH OF YOU
A practical guide to overcoming sex problems
Martin Cole and Windy Dryden

This essential guide for men and women is for those who are usually sexually confident, as well as for those for whom sex and anxiety go hand in hand.

Written by two highly experienced therapists this book presents the facts about sex and sex therapy in a readable and accessible style, offering practical and reassuring help.

PANIC ATTACKS
A practical guide to recognising and dealing with feelings of panic
Sue Breton

Panic attacks can ruin your life – but it lies within your power to overcome your fears. Sue Breton, clinical psychologist, researcher and former sufferer, shows you how to help yourself by recognising situations and symptoms which trigger an attack, understanding what type of attack you have and taking short term action to suit your personal needs.

The technique and advice given in this book will give you power over panic for good.

DIY PSYCHOTHERAPY
A practical guide to self-analysis
Martin Shepherd

Would you like to understand yourself better? Dr Shepherd draws on his long experience as a professional therapist to present this do-it-yourself approach to psychotherapy. Each chapter focuses on one aspect of human behaviour and concludes with a series of exercises designed to give you a clearer understanding of your own thoughts and responses.

Extremely practical and easy to follow, this book will enhance your enjoyment of life, and save you a fortune in therapist's fees!

To order any of these books direct from Vermilion (p+p free), use the form below or call our credit-card hotline on **01279 427203.**

Please send me

...... copies of **ALL IN THE MIND?** @ £8.99 each

...... copies of **PERSONAL THERAPY** @ £8.99 each

...... copies of **BE ASSERTIVE** @ £6.99 each

...... copies of **SEX: HOW TO MAKE IT BETTER FOR BOTH OF YOU** @ £8.99 each

...... copies of **PANIC ATTACKS** @ £8.99 each

...... copies of **DIY PSYCHOTHERAPY** @ £8.99 each

Mr/Ms/Mrs/Miss/Other (Block Letters)

....

Address...

....

....

Postcode.............................Signed...................................

HOW TO PAY

☐ I enclose a cheque/postal order for
£.............................. made payable to 'Vermilion'
☐ I wish to pay by Access/Visa card (delete where appropriate)
Card Number ☐☐☐☐☐☐☐☐☐☐☐☐☐☐☐☐
Expiry Date ☐☐☐☐

Post order to **Murlyn Services Ltd, PO Box 50, Harlow, Essex CM17 0DZ.**

POSTAGE AND PACKING ARE FREE. Offer open in Great Britain including Northern Ireland. Books should arrive less than 28 days after we receive your order; they are subject to availability at time of ordering. If not entirely satisfied return in the same packaging and condition as received with a covering letter within 7 days. Vermilion books are available from all good booksellers.